MW01593631

One Nation
Under God

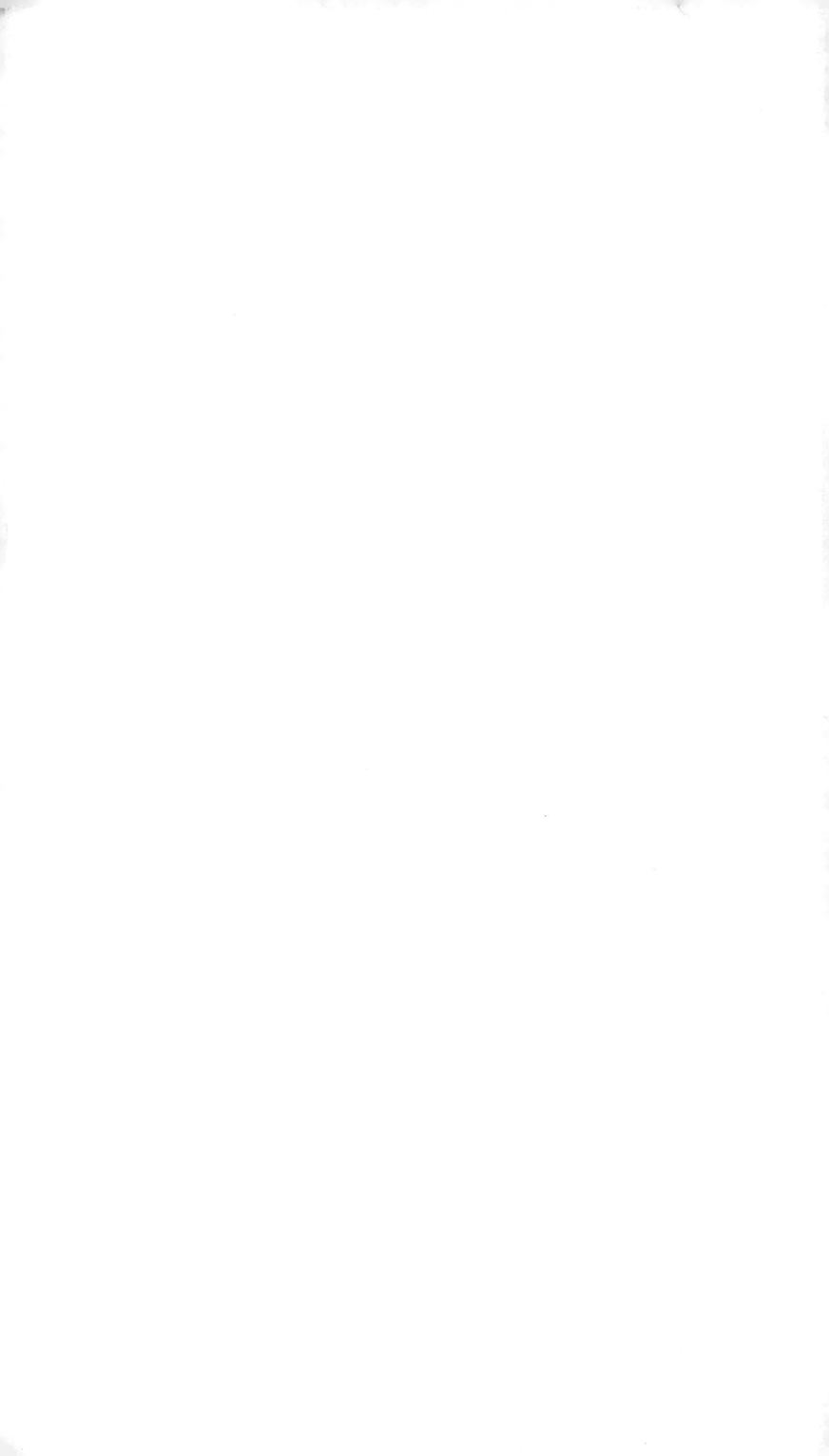

SMASHING
the GATES *of*
the **Enemy**
...through strategic prayers

Taiwo Olusegun Ayeni

Bloomington, IN 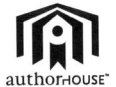 Milton Keynes, UK

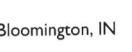

AuthorHouse™
1663 Liberty Drive, Suite 200
Bloomington, IN 47403
www.authorhouse.com
Phone: 1-800-839-8640

AuthorHouse™ UK Ltd.
500 Avebury Boulevard
Central Milton Keynes, MK9 2BE
www.authorhouse.co.uk
Phone: 08001974150

First published by AuthorHouse 3/28/2006

ISBN: 1-4259-2334-8 (sc)

Printed in the United States of America
Bloomington, Indiana

This book is printed on acid-free paper.

Rehoboth Bible Ministries Inc Publications
607 E. Abram, Suite One,
Arlington, Texas, 76010 USA
Tel:1-.(972) 602-1837
Tel:1- (972) 742-7365
Fax: 1-972-602-1837
Or
The Household of Faith Parish
The Redeemed Christian Church of God
5001 New York Avenue,
Arlington Texas, 76018, USA
Tel.:1-817-461-8857
Fax: 1- 817-676-9067
E-mail: taayeni@yahoo.com
Website: www.rehobothbministries.org

Dedication

I dedicate this book with great gratitude to the Almighty God who has found me worthy of use in His vineyard and poured his anointing on me. Unto Him I give thanks.

And to the oppressed, downtrodden and afflicted souls who have desired deliverance with passion for so long, arise and shine, for your light is come, the glory of the lord shall indeed rise on you in Jesus name. Amen.

Acknowledgements

That this book is published is because the Almighty God is merciful and full of glory, power and majesty. The devil tried all he could to stop this work at various stages of publication by hitting hard at the key personalities involved in the production of the book. The first in the series *"Fighting Your Way To Victory"* and this were supposed to be published simultaneously, but the devil hindered. However, this delay turned out together for good, as the merciful Lord opened unto us a door of mercy to do a proper re-arrangement of the chapters and increase the chapters from seven to ten.

In spite of the stiff opposition God raised men who willingly offered themselves to provide succor, and encouragement at the point when it seemed hopeless to go forward. While I was totally incarcerated, they did the running around to make this work a success. On top of the list is my amiable wife Dr. (Mrs.) Abidemi Olubisi Ayeni, Pastor and Sister Wole Ajayi, Pastor and Deaconess

Bisi Olowoyo, Pastor and Deaconess Dejo Oluwaniyi, Deaconess Taiwo Adekola, Pastor and Mrs. Isaac Ayodele Adeleke, Pastor and Deaconess Olaitan Olubiyi, Bros Taiye and Bayo Adekola. Worthy of mention also was the effort of Deacon Segun Otenaike, who as his own contribution carted all the materials used for printing the two series from Lagos to Ibadan.

Also special thanks go to Reverend Dr Moses Olanrewaju Aransiola who I gave so much hassles to write the forwards for both books in spite of his busy schedules. Sir, "May God continue to uplift you and perfect that which concerns you in Jesus name".

I cannot forget at this stage my Editor-in-Chief, Sister Olubusola Ajayi who in spite of all the oppositions raised against the work by the devil still pressed on to edit the various versions of this book at a great cost to her. I wish to appreciate her tireless, selfless and invaluable contributions, which included having to rewrite some portions of this book in order to give it a touch of class. She is indeed a good soldier of Christ who has endured hardness. I prophesy that you will surely overcome all obstacles in life in Jesus name.

I am greatly indebted to Pastor Wole Ajayi, the Area Pastor of Zion Assembly Parish of the Redeemed Christian Church of God, Ire-Akari, Lagos and Pastor Olaitan Agboola of The Lords Chapel, of the Redeemed Christian Church Gbagada for the use of their computer equipment for editing and printing of the original documents at various times.

Reverend Dr. (Mrs.) A. M. Oshodi who we fondly call 'Grandma', is sincerely appreciated for her motherly inspiration, fellowship, love, companionship, scholarly approach to the word of God in particular and various issues of life in general. Your contributions in cash and kind are deeply appreciated. Your desire to see the word of God fulfilled as it is written shall come to pass in your life and that of your children in Jesus name.

Lastly, my profound gratitude goes to my sweet Abidemi Olubisi Ayeni for all she silently did to make this a reality and to my children Rereloluwa (Son) and Oreoluwa (daughter) who at various times sat by me why I kept vigil behind my computer typing and editing the various corrections made on this book.

I really appreciate all of you, who have contributed in one way or the other. God bless and keep you till the coming of our king, the Lord Jesus Christ. Amen

Contents

Foreword

Gates are real and they limit, hinder, and prohibit men and nations from entering into their inheritance. But they can be lifted and uprooted. A gate can mean an opening, a place of entry and exit, a control point, a place of assembly or a parliament or in some other senses it means power or dominion. A gate is a place of Public concourse, a place to administer judgment. At other instances it can mean a barrier or a secret confederacy or a caucus gathering.

When the Lord Jesus Christ said: ***"I will build my church and the gates of hell shall not prevail against it"***. What He was saying indirectly is that the confederacy, assembly, dominion, or the barriers of hell would not prevail against His church. Thus, a gate is a place of power where decisions are made. For instance Daniel was a member of the Babylonian gate (court) - Daniel 2:48-49; while Modecai was also a member of the Medeo-Persian gate (Est.2:19-21).

The gate of hell is the house of assembly of hell, a place of the gathering of demonic powers. There they meet to take decision. It is the house of assembly of hell, a place of the gathering of demonic powers. There they meet to take decision to launch their attacks on the Body of Christ and all other interests of God on earth. That is what the word gate means. Every enemy we have as individuals and all enemies the Church has, have their seats at the gate. There is a group called the gates of hell. You must not let them prevail over you.

If we are to have lasting victory in life, business or ministry we must like the Lord Jesus Christ learn to take the battle to the gates of the enemy. Instead of going about His business and allowing Satan to choose the time and place of attack, Jesus took the initiative and went on the offensive after His baptism.

Before He announced His ministry agenda in the synagogue of Nazareth, before He called the twelve disciples, before He preached the sermon on the mount, before He walked on the sea, before He was transfigured, before He fed 5,000 people or raised Jairus daughter, the son of the widow of Nain or Lazarus from the dead, He knew He must engage Satan's kingdom in some crucial strategic-level spiritual warfare.

Jesus took the battle to the gate of the enemy. The place Jesus chose was strategic and significant He chose the word *eremos,* or "wilderness" which was known as 'Satan's territory'. The Dictionary of New Testament Theology says of eremos, the Greek word for wilderness or desert, that it is a place of deadly danger and of demonic powers - a type of gate, the entry point of Luciferic forces to the earth. Having won the battle at the gates, the rest of Jesus' ministry was as it were the gathering of the 'Spoils of war'.

This is precisely what the new book is all about – **STRATEGIC LEVEL PRAYER WARFARE**. Strategic prayers or warfare is simply a deliberate and sustained offensive prayers aimed at certain crucial targets (strongholds) the overthrow or destruction of which will bring an enormous release and break through in a life, neighborhood, city, or nation.

In this extra-ordinary book, the author Pastor Taiwo Ayeni who is one of my able ministry lieutenants and war strategist, has highlighted with a profound insight and wisdom the meanings of the Biblical word - gates, its implications on our lives, how to identify satanic gates and most importantly, how to deal with them.

This is a serious book from a very serious, loyal, teachable, intelligent, prayerful, national and kingdom conscious intercessor. Reading through the original manuscripts alone has done me a great good, and in Jesus mighty name, it will give to you and your prayer life a goodly increase too.

I commend this priceless book to the hands of the blessed Holy Spirit to use it, as an instrument of victory in spiritual warfare is His Church. May this book go around the world in Jesus name. Amen.

Rev (Dr.) Moses Olanrewaju Aransiola
President, Gethsemane Prayer Ministries Int'l
Ibadan, Nigeria.

Preface

I thank the Almighty God for bringing me across men, early in my Christian life, who assisted in laying a solid foundation for me in the areas of prayer, and spiritual warfare. Men who were willing to lay down their lives in order, for those under satanic affliction to receive their deliverance. Having traveled the length and breadth of the nation with them as a disciple learning under them, I have come to understand, through their teachings, the reason why men suffer, and how men could be delivered from bondage.

In addition to this, I have witnessed the operations of the kingdom of darkness in men's lives, in the course of my growing up. Many were and are still held bound by forces of darkness and satanic afflictions abound in many families, without any hope of deliverance.

The ignorance of men, and the leadership of the churches they belong to have compounded issues, and men have been forced to seek for help in wrong places. As a result some have been abused, tormented, used, harassed, and embarrassed. Some even die prematurely during the process, leaving the impression of a hopeless situation to the members of the family, who are also facing the same problem in life.

The weight of satanic afflictions, have seriously undermined the prayer lives of some, so much that they have been battered left, right and center, and the summary of their lives is they alternate between mountain and valley experiences. What makes matters worse is that the things that used to be walkover for them are now the subjects of prayers.

Having wandered from pillar to post in search of help, ashes have settled upon their prayer altars and many unfulfilled dreams, and shattered hopes are all they have to show for all their efforts. They have prayed. They have fasted. Yet nothing seems to have changed. Their situation is presently a tale of woes and except something is done fast, they may throw in the towel as frustration has set in. Those whom they used to counsel are now the ones they rely on for help. It is a terrible situation.

Beside the limitation in the place of prayers, they have lost the joy of their salvation. They desire a new experience, fresh exploits in the name of the Lord. They are sure there is hope, but how to get out of the mess they have found themselves in is an uphill task. This is the reason these series of lectures have been put together to show some light at the end of the tunnel or guarantee a ray of hope.

This is the second book in the series of work (Prayer school Manuals) originally titled *'The gates of Hell shall not prevail Parts I & II'*. While the first: *'Fighting Your Way To Victory – principles of victory over stubborn problems'* deals with the revival of prayer life, the second which is titled *'Smashing the Gates of the Enemy – through Strategic Prayers'* encourages the believer to engage in strategic spiritual warfare in order to unseat the powers of darkness limiting them from entering into their inheritance.

Basically, this book focuses on the operations of spiritual gates in men's lives. Many people have experienced limitations in life and have perceived a regular sequence of events passed down from generation to generation. They have experienced a history of failure at the point of success, and every attempt to go higher is thwarted by invisible barriers unknown to them.

The gates have defined the limits of the people's success and how far they can go in life. In order for them to break this barrier, there must be divine intervention. Such men require not only deliverance but the revival of their prayer lives in order to maintain the check on the forces of darkness operating in their lives.

The first step towards victory however, is to acknowledge the situation on the ground, through a personal and realistic assessment of ones life and stop pretending. Many today are nothing but hypocrites who suffer fools gladly. It is obvious to all that they are bound, yet they carry on as if nothing is happening.

This is the reason for the number of casualties being recorded in our various churches, as many die before their time because they fail to seek for help.

There is a need for the saints to arise in the place of prayers. We must go to the mountaintop to cry our hearts out until we receive deliverance, begin to walk in holiness, and possess our possessions. We must endeavour to fly high as the way of the eagle is in the sky. It is time to say no to sorrow, tears, and blood. Stand up to the oppressor, whip him and get the victory in Christ through prayers. The church of Christ must be built, and the gates of hell shall not prevail against it.

I pray that as you study this subject the Lord will help you to know Him in the place of prayer, become strong, and do exploits again in Jesus mighty name. Amen.

Chapter One
WHAT ARE SPIRITUAL GATES?

"…but Daniel sat in the gate of the king" (Dan 2:49)

Introduction

The subject of gates is crucial to our bid to enter into our inheritance in God in this end time. Many hopes have been dashed and lives rendered useless as a result of limitations imposed by the operations of gates. Even though several people have been shut out of their inheritance, they could neither explain nor comprehend the reason why. They have wandered from pillar to post in search of seemingly elusive solutions to their problems.

However, many people know little or nothing about gates of darkness and their operations. The few who do pay little or no attention to them. When confronted with inexplicable troubles of life they try to explain it away, yet the symptoms of continued affliction remain unchecked. A closer look at their situation reveals a soul under the stronghold of spiritual gates. The scriptures confirm the workings of spiritual gates, but sadly enough many are oblivious of their operations.

As we proceed, it is important to ask - what gate are we talking about? In the ordinary sense, there are many types of gate. Everyone is aware that physical gates are erected to control entry and exit into a house, block of apartments, office complex, city, town, or estate etc. However, the physical gates we see in those places mentioned are not actually the gates that shut men out of their inheritances. What many people have experienced, but could not give expression to is the fact that there are gates within the gates.

Beside the physical gates we see, there are spiritual gates at the entrance of every house, block of apartments, office complex, city, town, or estate etc. These are limitations that are experienced, and yet unseen, but their manifestations in the lives of some people are real as they reveal prolonged joblessness, delayed marriages, promotions, progress, and academic attainment. The contradictions they present show the hard working persons marking time, while the nonchalant are making rapid progress. That is the operation of gates for you. The good news however, is that the Lord declared in His word that: **"..the gates of hell shall not prevail"** against His church (Mt 16:18)

Physical Gates Defined

A gate is either a dual-leaf or single-leaf moveable barrier hinged to a fence or wall, which opens or shuts to grant or deny access to persons. In the simplest sense, it is a barrier designed to lock friends in, and enemies out. These kinds of gates are easily identified. While these gates are tangible, and familiar, there are other kinds of gates introduced to us in the Bible. Before we venture into them let us summarize the gates we are aware of. These are:

- Security gates of iron, brass and wood
- Men in authority as gates
- Spiritual gates – men who bear rule through spiritual powers.

Security Gates

We read from the Bible about gates of brass and bars of iron in Psalm Chapter 107 verse 16. There are also gates of wood. Gates are generally erected to provide security to the inhabitants of a home, office, city, town, communities, and nations. Gates are installed to lock out intruders. Some men voluntarily erected gates to shut themselves in to protect their lives and properties from petty thieves, rogues, assailants, burglars, and armed robbers.

The patriarchs in the Bible understood the importance of gates, and what they stood for. Hence in their prayers the constant refrain was: "*...and let thy seed possess the gate of those which hate them*" – (Gen 24:60).

We see the same repeated in the same book of Genesis when the angel of God prayed for him: ***"...and thy seed shall possess the gates of his enemy"*** (Gen 22:17).

Note that whoever controls the gate has dominion in his grasp. Lose control of the gate, and you are in big trouble, because this is akin to voluntary submission to plunder as unwanted intruder(s) can visit one with disaster.

In the book of Joshua Chapter 6 verse 1 we read how the people of Jericho effectively utilized the purpose for erecting gates.

"Now Jericho was strictly shut up because of the children of Israel: none went out and none came in".

Why did they shut their gates? The gates were shut because of the morbid fear of Israel's military prowess. The imminent threat that the nation of Israel posed against the nations around them spread terror like a wild wind. The people of Jericho have heard of the military exploits of Israel when coming out of Egypt, and how they have destroyed several powerful kings in battle. The story is best encapsulated in the words of Rahab the harlot in the book of Joshua Chapter 2 verses 9-10:

"And she said unto them, I know that the Lord hath given you the land, and that your terror is fallen upon us, and that all the inhabitants of the land faint because of you.

For we have heard how the Lord dried up the water of the Red Sea for you, when you came out of Egypt, and what you did to the two kings of the Amorites, that were on the other side Jordan, Sihon and Org, whom ye utterly destroyed".

Safety has always been the paramount reason for erecting gates in both old times and now. The current wave of violence and consequent insecurity in some parts of the world, has however led to extreme situation where people now erect barricades around themselves in the name of security.

Consider this scenario in a typical African home, say Nigeria, for example, you get to that house, press the bell, and the security man opens the gates. As soon as you step into the compound, you are confronted with another mini gates with several padlocks, and chains behind it. You press the bell, and your host opens several locks to admit you in and you pass through a door that before it was opened had three bars of iron behind it, to further fortify or reinforce it. Furthermore, the windows of the house, and every available exit point have burglary bars fixed into them.

Now imagine a fire incident or an attempt for somebody to rush a woman in labor to the hospital, you can be sure that before the various fortifications, and padlocks are removed at every point delivery would have taken place. When you think about it, some of our African friends are living in minimum, medium, or maximum-security prisons all in the name of security.

One cannot blame them because the terror unleashed by armed robbers, area boys and night marauders are too gruesome to be disregarded. Whether one likes it or not attention must be given to the situation, because the deadly operations of this demon infested imps are better imagined than being witnessed. May God deliver them from the hands of these ones.

However, the control of the gate is important as mentioned earlier on. This is because many people have come to learn of this in a very hard way. Some people because of the nature of their jobs have found themselves locked out of their homes by security guards. Even though they can see their house or apartment just a few meters away, yet the night guard who had been slain by the power of deep sleep could not hear the noise of frantic assault of flesh on metal. You find such men usually cursing and threatening fire and brimstone under their breath, **"If I catch this man today, I will make sure he is fired".**

It happened to me too several years ago in Nigeria before relocating to the United States of America. Of the eleven houses in the Estate I lived with my family, ours was the fourth from the main gate. Here I was returning from a preaching engagement (a vigil) in the early hours of the day, dog tired but confronted by the gate of my estate.

My reaction was spontaneous, and violently desperate as every part of my body was aching from lack of sleep. But I thank God for my wife, who happened to be a light sleeper, who saved me from the distress of the night. She heard the hooting of my car horn, alternated with my tired but anxious voice screaming in desperation. Strengthened by the possibility of danger outside the gate, I hit the gates so had that even the dead should wake up by the resonating sound of flesh banging on metal.

In spite of the one-man commotion squad, and the echoes of bedlam at dawn, our night guard did not wake up until my wife came out through our house gate to investigate the cause of the blare. On sighting me standing outside of the gate in that early hour, in a community where armed robbers operate with impunity cutting lives shot without caring a hoot; a sense of urgency took over. She walked about twenty meters to where the night guard was, to rouse him up from sleep, to go and open the gate. It took him a while to be fully awake enough to find the right keys to open the gates. It was a day of sweating mixed with anger at dawn. Thank God the gates were eventually opened.

Men As Gates

Besides the physical inanimate gate we are aware of, the Bible gives us insight into the fact that men can actually act as gates that shut others out of their inheritances. This is because of the powers such men have acquired over a period of time. Several references are made to men sitting in the gate. For example in Genesis Chapter 19 verse 1 we read: *"...and Lot sat in the gate of Sodom..."*

Also in Daniel Chapter 2 verse 49 the Bible has the to say about Daniel:

"Then Daniel requested of the king, and he set Shadrach, Meshach and Abednego, over the affairs of the province of Babylon: but Daniel sat in the gate of the king".

The question now is, does it mean both Lot, and Daniel are gate men? This is an interesting issue to investigate and verify. But notice that in both references the words used are:

"sat in the gate" and not *"sat at the gate"*

The interplay of words in this respect carries a deeper meaning than a man sitting at or by the gate. Even though they may not be termed to be gatemen, they may choose to sit at or by the gate to watch activities come in, and out. However, the issue here is that the gate in reference is the revealing of men who are **"power brokers"** or part of a **"decision making body"** such as a court of law or legislative body in their society.

The gate in reference is a place where justice, and legislative functions are being carried out in the governance of the people. The graphic example in the Bible that confirms this fact is found in the book of Isaiah Chapter 14 verse 31:

> *"Howl, o gate.."* (Referring to those in authority)
> *"Cry, O City.."* (Referring to the people)

A human gate is empowered by the people in a positive sense to represent them in government. He could be a president, governor, senator, and legislature etc. This representative, be he a president can act as a gate in many ways. For example, if both houses of government passed a bill restricting Japanese cars from coming into the United States, and the president affixed his signature to the bill, it becomes a law instantly. From that moment all Japanese cars will be gated from coming into the country.

In this case, what it means is that the body of government empowered by the people has taken a decision to shut out Japanese cars. The law enforcement agents will see to it that the legislative order is carried out as stated, and thereby enforce compliance. No matter what anybody does thereafter, as long as the law is in force, the gates will remain shut. It is only through the law court that this law can be challenged. The outcome of the case will then determine the later course of events whether the gates will be opened or not.

In a similar vein, a husband can act as a gate. If he issues an instruction that nobody should go out of the house after 9.00 p.m. or come in late after 10.00 p.m., it becomes a law in that house. He has the latitude to shut out night crawlers or neighbors who have no respect for time. He maintains order in his house. Anyone that flouts it is in trouble. The madam of the house as a faithful partner is a co-enforcer of such laws. This means she must be compliant, so that those that come in after the stipulated time are shut out.

A pastor can be a gate. He may decide to shut out incorrigible sheep that do nothing but cause division, rebellion and disaffection in the church. Even though excommunication is rarely used, where necessary the Bible permits it as means of correcting those who have fallen out of the way of truth, as we see in II John 10. ***"If there come any unto you, and bring not this doctrine, receive him not into your house, neither bid him God peed"***.

The Managing Director of a company can be one also. He may employ and may choose not to. He may decide later to fire and hire, it all depends on how he chooses to exercise the power reposed in him. He can shut out anybody who has been fired or any unwanted intruder. All he needs to do is to give instructions to that effect.

Since we have confirmed that gate is a place of decision-making, and dominion, anyone that has authority over you can act as a gate. A gate is in a nutshell is a person that has some level of authority and can exercise it either positively (for good) or negatively (for evil). He can intimidate, manipulate, indoctrinate, and dominate. Beyond this, gates can afflict and oppress. The evil gates cause bloodshed, sorrow, and tears. This leads us to the examination of spiritual gates.

Spiritual Gates

Spiritual gates in some cases are men who have unusual supernatural powers to afflict. These men are in high-level covenant relationships with demonic entities of darkness. Hence they are human beings with deadly spiritual capabilities. We see them in reference, operating in various ways in the Bible.

A typical example of the operations of spiritual gates, and the manifestation of wickedness expressed by these deadly beings, can be read in the gospel according to Mathew Chapter 22 verses 25-26, where we see how seven generations of family members were wickedly limited from receiving and enjoying God's gifts to them:

"Now there were with us seven brethren: and the first, when he had married a wife, deceased, and, having no issue, left his wife unto his brother. Likewise the second also, and the third, unto the seventh".

From this passage, we can see how spiritual gates limited seven (7) generations of people from entering into their inheritance. They all died without having fulfilled the covenant of God for their lives to be fruitful and multiply through procreation. They all died childless, while the woman had to go through the trauma of burying seven (7) husbands without any hope of deliverance.

There was a similar story of a woman who went through almost the same pathetic experience of frequent child losses. At every point in her conception, a satanic barrier or gate is raised before her to limit her from carrying the pregnancy through. My wife came across her while doing her Youth Service Corps postings, as a medical doctor, to one of the General Hospitals in Lagos, Nigeria. This woman had fourteen (14) pregnancies, and that were still born.

The interesting thing observed was the timing and regularity of her losses – all the pregnancies aborted at exactly seventh month. The spiritual gates that ruled over her situation apparently programmed the pregnancies to come down on the seventh month, and all fourteen did without fail. Mysteriously, fourteen children were lost through the operations of satanic gates.

In another situation, a woman lost four (4) children within a space of six years, and none of them lived beyond six hours! Incredible you may say, but it is true. Sadly enough both women mentioned suffered intensely in the hand of the devil because no one knew what to do. It was equally painful to know that the first woman was a believer, and member of a thriving fourth largest Pentecostal church in Lagos, with branches all over the states of Nigeria. In spite of her closeness to the possible expression of power, and operation of the Holy Spirit, those around her had little or no knowledge at all about the operation of satanic gatekeepers.

There was a third case, where a woman was forced to seek divine solution to her sudden inexplicable losses – two sons within six months. Her story was that within a few months of losing her children, pressures came from her husband's family to produce other sons to replace the two lost or else they would find another woman for him who could. She was confronted with this wicked ultimatum in the midst of her grief. The situation became so desperate that she was not able to hold down pregnancies for about three years after, yet the threat from her in-laws increased.

In the course of her travail, she was invited to a one-week prayer school organized by one of the churches in her community, with the hope of finding a solution to her problem. However, a few weeks before the prayer school, her husband who was a silent cooperator with the family informed her that the woman who would carry out his family's wish had been found, and he was traveling to the village to meet her. Before any damage could be done to her marriage, she pleaded with him to exercise patience and told him "Please give me till after the prayer school, if I do not give you a son, then you can go and marry another wife".

This was a challenge that faith drew out of her, in the midst of her terrible situation. Even though it was not convenient for her, she made sure she never missed any of the services during the program. It was during the counseling and deliverance prayer session that God visited her. When I had her story I was moved, and I prayed with her, commanding the roots of afflictions to be broken. In line with the true words of God that they that seek Him will find Him, this woman was delivered from powers of darkness.

After the prayer session, she vowed to call immediately her pregnancy passed seven months, and name the child Samuel if it was a son. She did as she promised on the eight month, and invited me on the delivery of the baby boy to name him Samuel. The birth of Samuel secured this woman's home from the oppression of gatekeepers.

Situations like these explain the reason why many people suffer, and bear no fruit despite hard work put into their business ventures. The limits and heights of success have been defined by the powers that be. These men control the lives of other men, and their future inheritance because they possess unusual supernatural powers. They have entered into covenants with death, and hell, so nothing seems to bother them (Isaiah 28:15).

It is a cartel that one must belong to in order to succeed. By so doing some find themselves in cults, and the result of this limitation or barrier is the reason why the wealth or the riches of the nation are concentrated in a few hands. If we must enjoy the move of God in our land and experience the breakthrough Jesus promised us, we must confront these gates of wickedness.

In order for the Church to enter into the inheritance of salvation, and enjoy all the benefits that go with it, our Lord had to deal with the gates of hell in Psalm 24 verse 7:

"Lift up your heads, O ye gates; and be ye lift up, ye everlasting doors; and the king of glory shall come in".

There is therefore a need to look inward, and make up your mind to do likewise. Ask yourself where the problem actually is, and do not explain it away. Take time off, settle down somewhere, and ask yourself serious questions. Be very objective and factual, detaching yourself from family emotion, and take a panoramic view of the family tree. Where there are cases of regular repeated afflictions along the family line, it is the indication of the operations of satanic overlords. You may then from this observation trace the origin of the problems, but asking elders in the family serious questions. Their response in this regards, will help you to know what to do next. God bless you.

FIERY DART PRAYERS

1. Let every veil preventing me from identifying the operations of gates in my life be uncovered.

2. I command all satanic limitations hindering me from advancing into my destiny be removed in Jesus name.

3. I desecrate every satanic altar raised against my family and I in Jesus name.

4. I cancel any barrier spiritual gates have erected against my prosperity in life in Jesus name.

5. I use the key of David to unlock every door shut against my progress in Jesus name.

6. I intercept with the shield of faith every satanic arrow shot against my family and I in Jesus name..

7. I erase with the blood of Jesus every invisible mark of failure satanic overlords have placed over my life.

8. Let my people who sit in darkness see the great light.

9. I receive grace for a turn around in blessings, prosperity, favor, and health in my life Jesus name.

10. I receive discharge and acquittal from the Lord, against satanic judgment in Jesus name.

Chapter Two
UNDERSTANDING SPIRITUAL GATES

"And Jacob awaked out of his sleep, and he said, surely the Lord is in this place; and I knew it not. And he was afraid, and said, how dreadful is this place! this is none other but the house of God, and this is the gate of heaven.". - Gen. 28:16-17

Introduction

Spiritual gates are men who are in covenants with evil powers, and have their backing to operate as satanic priest over altars of affliction. Hence, they possess unusual supernatural powers to afflict. Since we have confirmed that the gate is a place of decision-making and dominion, any one that has dominion over you can act as a gate. He can intimidate, manipulate, indoctrinate, and dominate. In addition gates can afflict and oppress. The evil gates cause sorrow, tears, and blood.

In the book **'The Secret of Breakthrough Prayers'** Reverend (Dr) Moses Olanrewaju Aransiola in Chapter 10 page 171 gave a wonderful and sound definition of gates, I quote:

*1 '....the gate simply means a place of assembly or a parliament or in some other instances it means power or dominion. At other instances it can mean a barrier or a confederacy or a gathering. When the Lord Jesus said, *"I will build my church and the gates of hell shall not prevail against it"* what He was saying indirectly is that the confederacy, assembly, dominion or the barriers of hell will not prevail against His church. Thus, a gate is a place where decisions are made. It is the house of assembly of hell, a place of the gathering of demonic powers. There they meet to take decision and launch their attacks on the Body of Christ and all other interests of God on earth. That is what the word gate means. Every enemy we have as individuals and all enemies the Church has, have their seats at the gate. There is a group called the gates of hell.'

Nobody is attacked by accident. Before you are attacked, may be in the dream, in the house, in the office or in the car, such decisions would have been taken somewhere before the physical occurrence............'

From the above definition, we can see that the subject of gates is all embracing and partial treatment of the subject is not sufficient to explain all there is to it. We are able to identify from the definition that a gate:

- is a place of assembly or parliament where decisions are made.
- means power or dominion
- is a barrier
- is a confederacy or gathering of demonic powers

The tremendous power gates possess, and the position they occupy in the society they belong becomes obvious. The hopes, and aspirations of many depend on them. The attacks men face in life whether in dreams or in the physical are attributed to the operations of gates.

Furthermore, we find an interesting affirmation of the above definition quoted in the book **Elders at the Gate** by Rev. Mosy U. Madugba in Chapter 5, pages 31 and 32 I quote:

> [2] 'The gates were an important part of any ancient city. They gave the only way of passing through the wall and were normally closed at night and were strengthened by bars of brass or iron. The gate is the name given to a very important place of concourse, partly because it was an open space, not usually found elsewhere in a city. Much of the business of the city was done there (Ruth 4:11).
>
> The word gate is sometimes associated with power, dominion or control. God promised and instructed Abraham that his posterity should possess the gates of their enemies, their towns, and their fortress, Gen 22:17. They should conquer them, and have dominion over them. The gates of death are the brink or mouth of the grave.

The above definitions are clear and self explanatory. When speaking about spiritual gates of significance, we would want to consider personal gates, home/family gates, compound gates, neigbourhood gates, city gates, local government gates, state or provincial gates, national gates, continental gates and global and world gates. Each of these gates should serve their purpose or else there will be problems.'

From the above quotation, we are also able to identify that a gate:

- is a barrier or a doorway
- is a place of concourse where decisions are made
- is sometimes associated with power, dominion or control
- also includes personal gates, home/family gates, compound gates, neighborhood gates, city gates, local government gates, state or provincial gates, national gates, continental gates and global and world gates.

Through this definition, we have identified several other gates coming into focus. In fact, the book reveals how your mouth, tongue, hands, eyes, sexual organs etc serve as gateways of afflictions. If you use them as instruments of sin serving the devil, you open up yourself for demonic oppression. However, the focus in this work is the operation of spiritual gates and how to deal with them.

Elders in the gate

There is a positive side to the subject of gates. While the gates of hell work tirelessly to hinder men from entering into their inheritance, there are elders in the gate that God has raised to confront the gates of hell.

Who is an elder? It is very important to clearly define who an elder is. These are the representatives of the gates of heaven. They are spirit-filled, demon-chasing and heavenly bound Christians, who have chosen to be transparent and live holy They are men who have been chosen by God to have a close walk with him, and thereby have controlling power over God's assigned territory. They bear rule through maintaining their covenant of life, and godliness with God.

These are men who have made up their minds to pay the price of service, holding forth the word of truth, with unalloyed faith in God and willing to risk their lives for the cause of Christ in their nation, community, city, town, village etc as the case may be. They are the friends of God.

Let us refer to the book **Elders at the Gate** by Rev. Mosy U. Madugba in Chapter 1, pages 1 and 2 for confirmation:

> [3] "When we speak of Christian Elders at the city gates we refer to men and women of God (not boys and girls) who are blood washed, sanctified and filled with the Holy Spirit. These must be men of integrity whose lives are dedicated to God as an offering in

righteousness. Often these are men who have by their personal knowledge and experience with God known the mind of God on general and specific issues and are committed to walking with God on a daily basis. They must be long enough in the faith to be spiritually mature and knowledgeable in the scriptures to teach others about our faith and the principles that represent the keys of the kingdom, and the manners and customs of the kingdom. They have lived long enough in the house that they know all the corners and can take a stranger around. They must be people whom we can say have been circumcised in the foreskin of their hearts. In whom various forms of superficialities, sensual coatings and childishness in spiritual matters have been cut off. Col 2:11, using the word of Paul to Timothy in 2 Tim. 3:17b "..they have been to a great extent thoroughly furnished unto all good works". After they have been purged of the things that are capable of reducing potential gold to clay and wood useful only for dishonorable tasks (2 Tim. 2:21).

They come from various professions; they have wisdom, which they have developed with age, reading, experience, exposure and wide interaction.

They could be Apostles, Evangelists, Prophets, Teachers, Pastors, and heads of denominations of ministries, successful businessmen or women, lawyers, active housewives. They could come from the Police or Military or Judiciary. They could be active government officials or retired persons who are no longer distracted by jobs outside the home."

It is clear that it is not just any person that can stand as an elder in the gate. There is a risk involved because he must be able to confront powers of darkness ruling over the community, city, state, nation etc as the case may be. He must have had wide experience in leadership, handling of spiritual matters and trained in the art of spiritual warfare. He must be an example unto others, one whom others wish to emulate his humility, transparency, holiness, and faith.

His home should be a reference point to others who desire leadership position in the body of Christ. He must be a thoroughly detribalized man, who is mature in all department of life. One who is totally sold out to the Lord and willing to pay the price of service no matter the cost. Having had divine call, separation and contact with God he is uniquely positioned to be God's man on ground in the community he finds himself. He is called to take charge as God leads him to fulfill His purpose here on earth.

The position of an elder is not such that a run-off-the-mill kind of person can fit in, as thoroughness, candor, discipline, boldness, and submission to God are necessary factors that make up an elder. Rev. Mosy U. Madugba in **Elders at the Gate** Chapter 1, pages 2 and 3 helps us to clarify the above assertion:

> [4] "They are not local church elders ordained by local assemblies with varying criteria for various reasons. The divine position of the city elders is older than the church. They have been and are still the strength

of any throne or monarchy. Even in the throne of God, He has twenty-four Elders. The place of a city eldership is not won by votes and is not supposed to be open for all. It is for those who over the years have maintained exemplary successful Christian lifestyle and leadership, whose testimonies concerning their marriages, business life, and activities in their local churches and native communities edify and inspire others to the glory of God.

Maturity in the faith attested to by all is the basic criteria for qualification....The spiritual tasks handled sometimes at the gates are not such that ignorant or young good church men should be exposed to. Why? Simply because these tasks involve strategic level spiritual warfare which requires spiritual stamina and discipline. As a man is, so is his strength. Battles are won or lost at these gates. So you do not bring people there to make them feel good and important. It is not a political gathering but solely spiritual."

That an elder must be ready at all times goes without saying. The call to battle most of the time is spontaneous and he must be strong to confront, contain challenges from whatever quarters, and sustain the victory achieved. He must however do this with diligence, and Holy Spirit guidance.

This reminds me of a man of God that God woke up in the dead of the night, and instructed him to proceed to the border of the town. He promptly dressed up in obedience without asking any question, and went as instructed.. On getting to the border he found eight (8) men about to carry a major sacrifice into the town. These men could not be seen with the physical eyes, God opened the eyes of the man of God, who promptly ordered them to stop.

As soon as they saw him, because they knew what he stood for in the community, they began to plead for mercy. They insisted that they had not come to deal with his church members, but those 'church goers' who carry the Bible, and do not know what they are doing. The man of God insisted that as long as he lived in that town, he was responsible for every soul there. This is confirmed in the book of Ezekiel:

"He cried also in mine ears with a loud voice, saying, Cause them that have charge over the city to draw near, even every man with his destroying weapon in his hand" (Ezek. 9:1)

He commanded them to go back to where they came from, but because they were neither supposed to stop nor speak to anybody as they carried the sacrifice of death, all the eight men died before the end of that year. So the elder in the gate came to the rescue because he was an elder whose spiritual eyes were opened.

In Israel in those days anybody that had a problem with another person went to the gate for redress. The elders sat in the gate to adjudicate on crucial matters that affected men's lives. That is why Deuteronomy 25:5,7 records that:

"If brethren dwell together, and one of them die, and have no child, the wife of the dead shall not marry

without unto a stranger: her husband's brother shall go in unto her, and take her to him to wife, and perform the duty of an husband's brother unto her.

And if the man like not to take his brother's wife, then let his brother's wife go up to the gate unto the elders, and say, My husbands brother refuseth to raise up unto his brother a name in Israel, he will not perform the duty of my husband's brother."

Boaz in Ruth 4:1, and verse 11 carried out this advice, when he wanted to have the hand of Ruth in marriage. The near kinsman who was supposed to take her refused to do so, because he did not want to mar his own inheritance. In accordance with the custom of that time the man plucked off his shoe and gave it to Boaz (v8). After this was done Boaz became the legitimate owner of Ruth. So in verse 11 we read:

"And all the people that were in the gate, and the elders said, We are witnesses..."

The elders solved the problem because they had been given the authority to do so. There are instances where elders in the gate become corrupt and wicked. This opens up the people to ridicule; shame, oppression, and injustice become the order of the day. There is no where to turn to in order to seek for redress because:

"They that sit in the gate speak against me;(Ps 69:12) *".... and their right hand is full of bribes"* (Ps 26:10).

The book of Amos 5:12 also confirms that the gates of the enemies: ***"...afflict the just, they take a bribe, and they turn aside the poor in the gate from their right"***. Who are the people used to mete out this heartless wickedness upon the people? These are those that sit ***"in the gate"***. They were supposed to guarantee the inalienable rights of the people but have turned their backs on them. They bring affliction upon the just, because they have been bribed to do so. The book in verse 10 goes on to reiterate the fact that these wicked people:

"....hate him that rebuketh in the gate, and they abhor him that speaketh uprightly"

Any one that is on the side of truth is hated with passion, and possibly gotten out of the way through high level politicking or get wasted through assassins bullets or prearranged accident. The living God has a harsh word for these people except they repent the following shall be their portion:

"Forasmuch therefore as your treading is upon the poor, and ye take from him burdens of wheat: ye have built houses of hewn stone, but ye shall not dwell in them; ye have planted pleasant vineyards, but ye shall not drink wine of them." (Amos 5:11).

God is not pleased when things degenerate to this point and bares His mind in Ps 82:2-4.

"How long will ye judge unjustly, and accept the persons of the wicked? Selah. Defend the poor and fatherless: do justice to the afflicted and needy. Deliver the poor and needy: rid them out of the hand of the wicked"

It is a big problem if elders cease from the gate as we also see in Lamentation 5:14: *"The elders have ceased from the gate...."*.

It usually results in a state of anarchy, as it happened in the time of Judges recorded in the book of Judges chapter 17 verse 6:

"In those days there was no king in Israel, but every man did that which was right in his own eyes".

What led to this situation? It was the sin of the fathers (Lam 5:7). As a result of this sin, the door was opened to the consequence of sin. Furthermore, prayerlessness and wickedness compounded the problem in the land at that time. Prayerlessness is cessation of prayers or a voluntary withdrawal from the place of communion with the God of your covenant. It is having an alternative to God's helping hands, and remembering him only in the time of trouble. It occurs when a man abandons fellowship or the love relationship with God.

This in essence means a man has issued a letter of divorce to God and warmly embraced Satan in a warm love relationship. It is an outright rebellion against God's command or instruction to pray. It is a confession, and confirmation that God cannot help you and so, you must sell your self cheap to Satan the enemy of God and the book of Judges 5:8 confirms that:

"They chose new gods; then was war in the gates...."

Therefore, great affliction befell the people and the following testimony was the fruit harvested from the sins of the fathers. Therefore:

"Servants have ruled over us: there is none that doth deliver us out of their hand. We gat our bread with the peril of our lives because of the sword of the wilderness. Our skin was black like an oven because of the terrible famine. They ravished the women in Zion, and the maids in the cities of Judah. Princes are hanged up by their hand: the faces of elders were not honoured. They took the young men to grind, and the children fell under the wood." (Lam. 5:8-13)

The people suffered so much because they did not take the battle to the gates. They allowed the enemy to take the initiative and spiritual warfare, which was supposed to be carried out against the enemy, was undermined, because of the guilt of sin. They abdicated the mountain of the Lord, the place of prayer, and the foxes took advantage of this:

"Because of the mountain of Zion, which is desolate the foxes walk upon it" (Lam. 5:18).

The crown of authority fell off their heads, their heart fainted, their eyes grew dim (verses 16-17), and several other unimaginable things that ought not to happen to the people of God afflicted them. Why? Because the foxes took over and plundered the people for leaving their flanks open.

This situation revealed the secret behind the familiar cry in the Songs of Solomon 2:15:

"Take us the foxes, the little foxes, that spoil the vines:.."

The foxes are in men's lives to kill, steal and destroy, and they did so maximally in the land of Israel, because they refused to arrest them. By the time the captives decided to arrest the foxes, it was too late. The damage had already being done and the Bible records that:

"The joy of our heart is ceased; our dance is turned into mourning" (Lam. 5:15).

What is God's ordained prescription to get men out of this rot? This we find enumerated in Amos 5:14-15:

"Seek good, and not evil, that ye may live: and so the Lord, the God of hosts, shall be with you, as ye have spoken. Hate the evil, and love the good, and establish judgment in the gate: ..."

Further to this God in very stronger terms reechoed this issue in the book of Zechariah chapter 7 verses 9 and 10:

"Thus speaketh the Lord of hosts, saying, Execute true judgment, and shew mercy and compassions every man to his brother: And oppress not the widow, nor the fatherless, the stranger nor the poor; and let none of you imagine evil against his brother in your heart."

With frank finality, the Lord reemphasized the issue in Zechariah chapter 8 verses 16 and 17:

"These are the things that ye shall do; Speak ye every man the truth to his neighbour; execute the judgment of truth and peace in your gates: And let none of you imagine evil in your hearts against his neighbor; and love no false oath: for all these are things that I hate, saith the Lord."

If the elders in the gate are able to adhere to this divine guidance, it shall be well with the nation and the pathway to breakthrough would be carved out. And the Lord's Christ will reveal Himself in our crisis as we are empowered to turn the battle to the gates.

FIERY DART PRAYERS

1.   Lift up your heads, O ye gates that I may enter into my inheritance in Jesus name.

2.   I scatter in the name of Jesus the assembly of evil men presiding over my case.

3.   I use the word of God as a fire to burn to ashes any altar of affliction raised against my success in the name of Jesus.

5. I cancel any barrier spiritual gates have erected against my prosperity in life in Jesus name.

5. I use the key of David to unlock every door shut against my progress in Jesus name.

6. I break in the name of Jesus every existing covenant legally binding my lineage to poverty and affliction.

7. O ye everlasting doors, I command you to be opened so that I may come in to possess my possessions.

8. O Lord! Let my people who sit in darkness see the great light and gravitate towards liberty in Jesus name.

9. O Lord, expose every ploy of Satan to bind me in ignorance in Jesus name.

10. I receive discharge and acquittal from the Lord, against satanic judgment gotten against my lineage from satanic courts in Jesus name.

Chapter Three
THE OPERATIONS OF SPIRITUAL GATES

"Then said I, What come these to do? And he spake, saying, These are the horns which have scattered Judah, so that no man did lift up his head: but these are come to cast out the horns of the Gentiles, which lifted up their horn over the land of Judah to scatter it" (Zech. 1:21)

Introduction.

It is pertinent for us to now identify the operation or workings of gates. How do they operate? Why are they successful in their attacks against men? What is the secret behind their potent power? Why do they prove so difficult to identify and subsequently dealt with? We saw earlier in this book, how seven men in the gospel of Mathew Chapter 22 verse 25-26 had their destinies terminated, and they all died childless. Let us briefly identify the operations of spiritual gates below.

i) They Take Permission To Strike

The book of Job Chapter 1 verses 6 to 10 reveals to us the operations of gates. The council in heaven was at a meeting presided over by the gate of heaven himself (God) and there came the gate of hell (Lucifer) to intrude in order to seek for permission to afflict Job. This he got easily, because Job was busy praying for his untutored children not to sin against God. The Bible says:

"And his sons went and feasted in their houses, every one his day; and sent and called for their three sisters to eat and to drink with them." (v4).

Their actions degenerated from ordinary feasting into drinking and surfeiting. Their father neither cautioned nor trained them in the way of the Lord, but busied himself praying for them not to sin. He spent all his time praying on behalf of children, and offering sacrifices of repentance rather than thanksgiving and righteousness,

"...for Job said, It may be that my sons have sinned, and cursed God in their hearts. Thus did Job continually" (v5).

That which he feared came upon him, because he shirked his responsibility as a father. The affliction of Job came as a result of closed heaven praying. Despite his commitment to continuous prayer, he did not pick the signal of an impending attack. The discussion of

Lucifer with God was quite revealing as we can see in verse 10. He emphasizes the fivefold protection over the life of a believer. These are:

- Has not thou made an hedge about him?
- And about his house?
- And about all that he has on every side?
- Thou hast blessed the work of his hands,
- And his substance is increased in the land.

Even though the above facts were clearly obvious to the devil, Job did not know and he was anxiously offering sacrifices without putting his house in order. His conduct and that of his children opened him up for the fourfold attack the devil visited on him (v13-19). What was the reaction of Job to these attacks?

He became philosophical instead of reacting with violent prayers:

"And said, Naked came I out of my mother's womb, and naked shall I return thither: the Lord gave, and the Lord hath taken away; blessed be the name of the Lord." (v21)

This is a lie of the devil. The devil stole from him and he philosophically attributed it to God. What an ignorant reaction! This was what gave the devil the audacity to strike him again in chapter 2:1-8. The gates blinded him, wasted his loved ones and investments in life. The man Job completely surrendered the initiatives to the gates of hell and he indeed paid dearly for it.

We however, a different attitude in Hezekiah, whom the gate of heaven (God) had given death sentence but took the matter to God in prayers. He refused the death sentence passed on him and:

"…. turned his face to the wall, and prayed unto the Lord…" (II kings 20:2).

This man refused to be philosophical. He was realistic in his cry so that the Bible recorded that:

"… Hezekiah wept sore" (v3).

The interesting thing here was that the prophet of God had not even left the premises of the king's palace before God answered his cry. The emphasis of God in His message to Hezekiah were: *"…. I have heard thy prayer, I have seen thy tears: behold I will heal thee…"* (v5).

How I wish men would receive this and act in faith against any judgmental move of powers against their lives. A sister, who is a nurse by profession, was bitten on her right leg by a cat in her dream. She woke wondering why it had to happen. Sometime later the leg got swollen, in spite of the prayers said over the leg. By the second day she was totally incarcerated, as she could not move about. It was at this point that her Pastor, who was worried about her condition, interviewed her further on what actually happened. She narrated in clear details, how a cat bit her right leg.

On hearing this account, the pastor was inspired to pray over the leg, commanding that the arrows shot at her, be returned back to the sender. Within a few days, the right leg of the matron in her hospital (her sworn enemy) began to swell up. This incident revealed the sender of the arrows. Deliverance came through strategic level praying and dealing with the root of the attack.

ii) They Strike on the Basis of Legality

The interesting thing to note, is that the gates of hell usually strike on the basis of legality, that is, they obtain judgment against an individual, as we saw in the case of Job, before they attacked him. They draw a man out of the hedge before they strike. They put a man in bondage based on the sins of the fathers, after they have dragged him to Satan's court where they get judgment against him or his family. On this basis, his punishment becomes perpetual except there is divine intervention. However, the book of Zephaniah 3:15 states that: *"The Lord hath taken away thy judgments, he hath cast out thine enemy:"*

This is reassuring as we confront the gates of hell to proclaim our liberty. The children of God seem to lack this knowledge, judging by the way the enemy has succeeded in the plundering and spoiling of lives.

A brother became mentally deranged as soon as the sister he proposed to gave him a positive answer. On prayerful investigation, it was discovered that the sister was received from water spirits and her mother had promised them that she would not get married. Prayer of deliverance was carried out: repentance, renouncement, and rejection of the promise were made and the yoke of oppression was broken. The legal ground that Satan had to afflict her and her life partner was dealt with and they were happily married thereafter following a successful Christian courtship.

iii) They Operate On The Basis Of Covenants

Several parents have innocently entered into a covenant of protection with Satan. This could be a blood, drink, or meal covenant. As long as this covenant exists, it must be serviced with the usual tokens or sacrifices offered to the gods of the covenant. Where the family reneges on the covenant, disaster will strike. The covenant remains binding for life except the family renounces, rejects, and breaks it. If this is not done, Satan will continue to have easy access to the family under oppression.

For example, the covenant requires the shedding of blood and it has not been carried out for a long while, the devil simply begins to draw blood directly from the womb through abortion, excessive menstrual flow or fibroid affliction that would elicit a heavy flow of blood that would distort the menstrual cycle of the person(s) involved.

In some cases, the blood is drawn through assassin's or armed robbers bullet, and accidents of various types e.g. car, kitchen knife, shaving blade cuts, finger nail cuts, tripping over obstacles, hitting one's foot against objects or falling down from heights etc. The major reason for the attack is to draw blood, the means by which it is done does not matter.

iv) Satanic Altars Back Them Up

Powerful satanic altars also back them up. The sacrifices you see on footpaths, and at road junctions, markets, shrines, hilltops, or mountainous terrain, water bodies or at the seaside are functional altars servicing the covenants with the gates of hell. Through these gates entities of darkness have passage to hold meetings in demonic cities in the sky, big baobab trees, under the earth, rivers and the sea.

These are satanic altars as well as gates of hell, where decisions over men's lives are taken, and some inheritances are destroyed or altered as the case may be. These altars are focal points for trafficking of spirits or entry points of spirits into the earth. A positive example is described in the book of Genesis Chapter 28 verses 16 to 18:

"And Jacob awaked out of his sleep, and he said, surely the Lord is in this place; and I knew it not.

And he was afraid, and said, how dreadful is this place! This is none other but the house of God, and this is the gate of heaven. And Jacob rose up early in the morning, and took the stone that he had put for his pillows, and set it up for a pillar, and poured oil upon the top of it".

The action of Jacob here in effect raised an altar unto the God of his covenant. In verses 12-15 he saw a ladder with angels ascending and descending on it (this is trafficking of spirits). Here God entered into a covenant of blessing with him, and this revelation and covenant informed his raising of the altar to God.

v) They Thrive on Ignorance and Atmosphere of Sin

If we must enjoy the move of God in our land, and experience the breakthrough Jesus promised us, we must confront these gates of wickedness. Even our Lord had to deal with the gates of hell in order for the Church to enter into the inheritance of salvation.

"Lift up your heads, O ye gates; and be ye lift up, ye everlasting doors; and the king of glory shall come in.

Who is the king of glory? The Lord strong, and mighty, the Lord mighty in battle.

Lift up your heads, O ye gates; even lift them up, ye everlasting doors; and the king of glory shall come in. Who is this king of glory? The Lord of host, he is the king of glory" (Ps. 27:7-10)

Sadly, enough the enemy has taken the battle to our gates. The manifestation of this is the inner wrangling going on, unhealthy rivalry, worldliness of the worst kind, covetousness, love of money, infidelity, and impurity that we see all around us. Our youths in their exuberance, under the guise of liberty of the spirit, have indulged in these vices beyond our wildest imagination.

There is a need to look inward, and ask ourselves where the problem actually lies. Why am I limited? Why has my business failed? Why did I fail my papers? Why has my marriage never worked? Why do I always have broken engagements? Why is promiscuity so rampant in the Church?

Where one of these is your situation, my friend the gates are at work in your life. It could be familiar gates, where only you in the family are affected. It could be ancestral gates, in which case the majority of the family is suffering limitations. The other extreme is when the whole community is shut out of their blessings; this is a territorial gate at work. Territorial altars backing the territorial gates generate powerful satanic powers, which produce a covering of darkness over that territory or community:

"The people that walked in darkness....' and '... they that dwell in the land of the shadow of death," *(Is. 9:2).*

Where this is in operation, the community experiences wickedness, immorality (prostitution, sodomy etc), untimely death, poverty, high crime rate, murder, and gross underdevelopment.

For some of us, it is something that we would like to wish away, but the truth is that except it is confronted we will not move forward. This is sad because the intention of the Master is that the battle of the last day should be carried out within the gates of the enemy. The initiative should come from us and we must set the pace for battle, anything less will spell our doom.

The truth is that, when God's altar(s) e.g. Church, house fellowships, or praying families or groups are operating in that area, a positive wave of God's glory ought to begin to manifest. It will seem to an on-looker that from the present happenings in the Church, we have disappointed the Lord, but the truth is that the Church will rise up again because:

"After two days will he revive us: in the third day he will raise us up, and we shall live in his sight.

Then shall we know, if we follow on to know the Lord: his going forth is prepared as the morning; and he shall come unto us as the rain, as the latter and former rain unto the earth" (Hos. 6: 2-3).

God is going to strengthen a group of mature people that will exhibit a high level of understanding, while turning the battle to the gates. These ones would be tested hands that had been discipled by the Elders in the gate.

As mentioned earlier when dealing with the subheading **Elders in the gate**, it is not just any person that can engage in dealing with the gates of the enemy. This is because of the risk involved. But the men we are discussing about would have made up their minds to pay the price of service, and hold forth the word of truth, with unhindered faith in God. They would be willing to risk their lives for the cause of Christ in their nations, communities, towns, villages etc as the case may be because *"Thy people shall be willing in the day of thy power......"* (Ps 110:3).

They would deal with the gates of the enemy, determine the course of the affairs of their nations, speed up the pace of the deliverance of the land, and wipe off the covering of darkness covering the face of the people.

Furthermore, they will restore sanity in the geographical areas wherein they live. Hence, the operations of gates, which make the community to experience wickedness, inexplicable community clashes, unstable marriages and high level of immorality (such as homo-sexuality, lesbianism, prostitution, bestiality etc), untimely death, poverty, high crime rate, murder and gross underdevelopment shall be eliminated with time. This is because the altars of God that have been raised in those areas will produce positive wave of God's glory so that:

"...thou mayest say to the prisoners Go forth; to them that are in darkness, shew yourselves...." (Isaiah 49:9).

FIERY DART PRAYERS

1. I halt every operation of satanic gates over my life in the name of Jesus.

2. In the name of Jesus I scatter the inner caucus of evil men, working against my progress.

3. I command the fire of God to burn the assembly of wicked men limiting me in life.

4. I release fire and brimstone upon every covenant enforcer, limiting my lineage from going forward.

5. I command every gate shut against my family to be opened now in Jesus name.

6. I neutralize all unknown agreements between my village, town or city with satanic gatekeepers in the name of Jesus.

7. Spirit of the living God, I resist every legal ground that my ancestors had given satanic powers to rule my lineage and proclaim the Lordship of Jesus over my family and I.

8. I repent, reject, and renounce any unknown covenants binding my family to poverty and failure.

9. I command fire and brimstone to fall upon the priest and the altar of sacrifice raised against my progress.

10. I receive discharge and acquittal from the Lord, against satanic judgment gotten against my lineage from satanic courts in Jesus name.

Chapter Four
THE CHARACTERISTICS OF SPIRITUAL GATES

"In that day shall the Lord of hosts be for a crown of glory, and for a diadem of beauty, unto the residue of his people, And for a spirit of judgment to him that sitteth in judgment, and for strength to them that turn the battle to the gate." - Isaiah 28:5-6

Characteristics of Gates

In order to carry out the relevant warfare strategy against the gates of hell and possess the land, you must understand the workings of gates, their operations and their characteristics in general. As discussed earlier, gates are evil men that grant access to spirits through the altars they have erected. These altars are entry points for spirits that control the communities over which they rule.

These spirits have given these men power to rule and that is the reason why you see certain men surviving various changes of government, whether it is military or civilian. When they assume power, they rule by sorcery, and depend heavily on the counsel of their satanic priests. Their influence is strongly felt in government, especially where certain crucial decisions have to be taken. It is whatsoever the gates favor that usually gets approved for implementation.

If you closely observe, there were times in which government could have adopted a position on an issue, and then suddenly you would see it backing out of that decision. Most of the time when it happens the gates have moved in to effect that change. Even though this decision may not be popular with the masses nobody will raise any alarm. The reason is the bewitching power that has been unleashed on the people. In some cases where an alarm is raised it is quelled by force, because they have their men in position, everywhere that matters.

Being thoroughly fortified positionally, financially, and spiritually they have available to them unlimited use of power and access to the nation's resources. This they plunder at will, and use to perpetuate themselves in office. Their presence in government brings the nation under the covering of darkness. This is why even right men with good intentions take wrong decisions. Their good works are turned to evil because of the pile of altars raised by successive leaderships.

This situation brings forth an effulgence of negative glory constituting a cloud over the nation with the resultant effect that men turn their backs on the word of God. Evangelism becomes difficult, men resist the doctrine of God, and the land cannot be possessed. It will take divine intervention to overcome them in order to possess the land for the Lord Jesus Christ. Let us now briefly itemize their characteristics.

i)   ***They are Powerful People Who Hold on to Power by Force*** - One common thing you notice about gates is that they are always in power at the community, local government, state and national levels, irrespective of the type of government ruling. It is not that they are particularly good or their presence is beneficial to the people, it is the superior spiritual advantage they possess that is at work.

They are there continually to protect their interests, satisfy the unseen and unknown (to the public) demands of the inner caucus of evil men. They survive several changes in ruler-ship and are recycled at will to the chagrin of the people to whom they have been exposed as non-performers.

Even at the traditional level, members of spiritual gates are installed as traditional chiefs or overlords etc against the wishes of their people. This obvious act of injustice has led to riots or clashes in many communities in Africa, and has brought untold hardship on the people because:

".... of the error which proceedeth from the ruler: Folly is set in great dignity..." and "...servants (sit) upon horses, and princes walking as servants upon the earth" (Eccl.10:5-7).

The people are cheated of their rights when the wicked rules.

ii) *They are Backed by Strong Covenants -* The satanic covenant these men have entered into guarantee their rapid rise in society, and in some cases, they exercise unrestrained authority. It is when you have personal contact with them that you can experience how they carry themselves. One may not be wrong to say that they act like gods, who are without feeling for humanity.

The book of Isaiah 28:15 provides us with an insight into why they do this. It is because they:

"...have made a covenant with death, and with hell..."

This covenant is the bedrock of their false hope and arrogance, and indeed the confidence with which they plunder whatsoever society they belong to. You ask yourself, what can make them afraid if they are in friendship with death and hell. Nothing seems to scare them. They are vicious, ruthless, and cruel.

iii) *They are Fetish and Rule by Sorcery -* The lives of these men totally depend on fetish sacrifices from which they bear rule. Since they are aware of the power backing them, they oppress the people like Sisera with his chariots oppressed Israel for twenty (20) years (Judges 4:3).

However, we thank God that the very spiritual instrument of oppression deployed by Sisera was manipulated to fight against him through the strategic level prayers of Prophetess Deborah. The book of Judges chapter 5 verse 20 reveals that:

"They fought from heaven; the stars in their courses fought against Sisera."

The secret here is that Sisera was a stargazer and through the manipulation of the heavenly bodies he had ruled the people for twenty years. This power was broken through the prophetic prayers of Deborah.

The book of Ezekiel 8:16 also reveals how elders in the city worship the sun, with their backs turned to the temple of God.

"And they brought me into the inner court of the Lord's house, and, behold, at the door of the temple of the Lord, between the porch and the altar, were about five and twenty men, with their backs toward the temple of the Lord, and their faces toward the east: and they worshipped the sun toward the east."

These were twenty-five (25) men that were supposed to be the 'Elders sitting in the gate' and ensuring righteousness and truth. What a disappointment? It does not make sense to think you can serve God, and the devil together, you have to choose who you wish to serve - one has to give way. Even their wives were not left out of this evil venture. They burnt incense to the queen of heaven (Jer. 44:15-19).

The desire to know, and sustain the future through fetish means is so prevalent in many African societies so much that this dangerous trend has also infiltrated the Church. People just desire instant results that they can see or feel. The political leaders are not left out of this bad business. They in fact spearhead these satanic consultations and their marks are already all over the land through all forms of satanic sacrifices, and offerings. We have several examples revealed in Nigeria, where through confessions of associates, how former military rulers imported marabous, who prescribed endless fetish sacrifices, in order to perpetuate themselves in office. The marabous recommended a lot of human sacrifices that brought upon the nation the blood of innocent people crying for vengeance.

One in fact had twenty-four (24) of them divided into three equal groups, each group praying eight hours of enchantments in three shifts for twenty-four hours every day for many years. But when God's judgment came, He hit them: ***".... upon the cheek bone..."*** (Ps 3:7), and prevented them from their enchantments and killed the wicked in spite of the heavy security network around him.

*iv) **They Operate Better at Night** -* The coalition of wicked men use the cover of the night to operate. The fate of many is sealed by very few in the deep of the night. This period is conducive to them because it is the time when men sleep. Many sleep at night only to wake up, and discover some dramatic changes in the situation of their lives and nation. In many instances, the plundering of lives, resources and wealth of nations are done at night "***...while men slept...***" (Mt 13:25).

*v)   **They are Proud and Arrogant People** -* The feeling that they are born to rule and reign is the erroneous foundation of their attitude. Being descendant of several generations of wealth, many things are taken for granted. Whether the wealth has clean foundation or not does not matter, they flaunt it anyhow. They have no scruples and will do anything to remain in control of their stinking wealth. The book of Isaiah gives an accurate description of these people. They are referred to as the:

*"**crown of pride**"* (Is 28:1, 3) and "*.. **scornful men, that rule this people.**"* (Is 28:14).

You can easily identify them in almost all arms of government, private sector, religious circles, and the society at large. What they do not know is that, the summary of their lives is that their:

"***...glorious beauty is a fading flower...***" (Is 28:1).

I remember the incident during the second republic in Nigeria, when people began to complain about the suffering of the masses. One of the ministers, who was notorious for his pride, arrogantly asked journalist what they meant by saying people were suffering? He asked further whether they had seen anybody eating from the dustbin. Where is this man today? He has faded away. That is the portion of the wicked.

vi) They Belong to Several Power Groups – Many of them belong to more than one power groups to secure their stay in power and thus become accessories to the covering of darkness that afflicts the society. While they have special places in the church or mosque as the case may be, they have membership chairs in secret societies where they actively participate. An example is described in the book of Ezekiel where symbols of various cults were portrayed on the wall with:

> *"...every man in the chamber of his imagery."* (Ezek. 8:7-12).

This means they lined up or took position behind the cults they represented. These were not ordinary men in the society. They were leaders of thought which included seventy elders, and others who:

> *"...devised mischief, and give wicked counsel in this city"* (Ezek 11:1-2).

vii) They Possess Double Personality and Unusual Ability to Lie - Spiritual gates possess an uncanny ability to lie and perpetrate falsehood. Of course when Satan their father speaks the Bible declares that lying is his native language, and he is the father of all liars. Wherever they rule the nation is built on a foundation of lies and falsehood:

"...for we have made lies our refuge, and under falsehood have we hid ourselves" (Is 28:15).

One of these men, a military despot ruled the Nigeria through lies for eight years till God in his infinite mercies delivered the people from his hands, by causing him to step aside. His tenure saw billions of Dollars wasted on a transition programs, that he knew would never work, and yet he tricked many people including his closest associates into penury, and outright destruction.

viii)They are Violent and Terribly Wicked People
- When they are in power they do everything imaginable to ridicule their subject and trample them into subjection. We saw the example of Pharaoh in Egypt (Ex 5:1-9) and the insult meted to Ahab by Ben-hadad (I kings 20:1-12). When confronted by superior force, however, their weakness is easily exposed. They usually deploy subtlety to overcome their predicament or find a way of quick escape because they are afraid to die (I kings 20:31-34).

They are terribly wicked people who neither forgive nor forget. Their wickedness is usually borne out of the repercussions they will suffer at the hands of their master if they fail in their wicked assignment. In Satan's kingdom there is no pity, and lives have no value.

ix) *They Cannot be Placated* - The basic motto of gates in their operation is **'Winner takes all'.** Where they concede any ground, it is because they are waiting for a better opportunity to hold their opponent at the jugular. Nothing will stop them until they reach their goal. The more you try to appease them, the more you put yourself at their mercy, and they have no milk of kindness at all.

Such was the case of a maximum despot, who made everybody believe that he was a fool and did not desire power. Almost everybody felt that he was not interested in power, because he was a soldier to the core, and that he would soon leave. How wrong his analysts were! Even the church fell for his tricks as several prophecies followed in tow to reassure brethren with respect to the man's person, and divine assignment!

The man capitalized on everybody's error of judgment, and disarmed the politicians as well as the masses. He tactfully won the favor of those who mattered, in spite of the clamor of a few journalist, and Human Rights group against handing over power to him. They warned us to watch out, because they read through his tricks and were not willing to fall for them.

A president-elect who had a political romance with him, in the hope of taking over power after things normalized was warned with the comment that he was riding on the back of a tiger, and that if he was not careful he would end up in the belly of the tiger – and that was exactly what happened.

The maximum despot gradually maintained his hold on power and turned the heat on his former suitors. By the time the politicians realized what they were into, the error had become fatal, as some lost their lives in the struggle, some were incarcerated, and others scurried into exile. It was a taste of hell for everybody as long as the man lived, but thank God for divine intervention that delivered the nation from the valley of the shadow of death.

In II kings 18:13-16, there is the Biblical example of how the wicked king of Assyria visited King Hezekiah with all sorts of insults until God intervened. The king tried to placate the king of Assyria by giving him all the silver that was found in the house of the Lord, the treasures of the King's house and even cut off the gold from the doors of the temple and the pillars.

Yet, he still sent his messengers to search his house and take whatsoever they found in his house. He went further to harass the people, and tormented them with psychological warfare. Everybody was terribly stressed until God intervened (II kings 18:17-37;19:1-5,14-15). He just could not be placated.

x) ***They are also in Religious Circles and always Support the Status Quo*** - They are like the Pharisees of old who withstood Jesus and made every attempt to frustrate his ministry. These are the advocates of cultural awareness or revival in the church, where men of the occult openly thrive, and are given prominent positions. Everything possible is done to maintain the status quo. They oppose vehemently any new move of God in their church and insist on the tradition of their fathers. Because of the enormous power they possess, they hit hard at any thing that wants to upset the balance, and in doing so they use a sledgehammer to kill a fly and cause damage of eternal consequence.

Damage such as legislation that hinders the preaching of the gospel in public places, placing restriction on foreign ministers who may wish to hold meetings in the country; and also placing restrictions on the use of government facilities for religious purposes are secretly instigated by them in order to maintain the status quo.

xi) ***They Hinder God's Plan or Work*** - The fact that they have access to power has put them in confrontation with God's plan. In Ezekiel 8:5-6 they erected an image of jealousy simply to drive God away from his sanctuary (house) and got God angry by being at ease:

"..for I was a but a little displeased, and they helped   forward the affliction." (Zech 1:15).

Consequently they hindered God's plan of blessing the people and the nation. God however, allowed a way out through prayers of repentance in order for the blessings (cities to be built) to come through His abundant mercies. (Zech 1:16-17).

xii) *They Promote Rebellion against God through Introduction of Cultural Revivals* - The introduction of this cultural reawakening is intended to put the nation or community under the covering of darkness. They encourage the promotion of fertility rites, female circumcision, incisions, tribal marks and body tattoos, initiation of babies, manhood or female-hood rites, and maintenance of traditional names etc These negate God's laws. (Leviticus 19:4,26-28; Deut 18:9-12), but they go ahead and do it all the same.

What they call cultural reawakening is Satan's ploy to pollute the nation and its people, and bring them under the covering of darkness (Is. 9:2). During these festivals, sacrifices and new covenants are made thus taking the people deeper into bondage and hindering God's blessing upon them.

xiii)*Ungodliness Thrives Around Them* - Their conscience is seared, and they can descend to any level of depravity to achieve their goal in life. It is common knowledge that some even turn their daughters into prostitutes to win contracts or as baits in a bid to blackmail their weak enemies.

"Do not prostitute thy daughter, to cause her to be a whore..." (Lev. 19:29).

Others include business-related and judicial murders, mayhem, arson, political cleansing, advance fee fraud (a.k.a. 419), and immoralities of all kinds.

xiv) ***They Raise Attacks on the Servants of God and the Church*** - These people are behind some of the scandals, and rumors raised against men of God, who refuse to compromise their stand. They have their men in the press or media houses whose mandate is to seek for any scam that may damage the reputation of men of God or the Church and publish it. They do this with so much skill that even the Christian community believes it, and also helps them to spread it bringing so much damage to God's servant, and His Church.

xv) ***They Are Negative Role Models*** - When you go to government functions, society weddings and other types of social gatherings the kind of dresses you see on parade portray the moral state of the society.

You need to see the scantily dressed Jezebels, and their paramours on parade, around the corridors of power. They come in all shapes, and colors in their mini skirts or transparent traditional gears swinging their hips, rolling their eyes, and attracting attention in order to draw the weak minds into the pit of mass destruction.

The TELL Magazine of April, 23 2001 titled 'A Revealing Trend' on page 66 captures it all:

> [1] 'Over the years, traditional attires gradually started giving way to western style of dressing. There were shirts, trousers, suits, gowns, skirts and blouses surfacing into the Nigerian fashion world. Of course, many Nigerians welcomed these outfits. They yearned to look like the film stars they saw on television and models in magazines. Today, many have resolved to go out half-naked in the name of fashion. Teenage girls, particularly have thrown the word 'modesty' into the bin, walking the streets in clothes like bare-back gowns, spaghetti strap tops, see-through outfits, tight trousers and skirts. These outfits which expose all, leave very little to the imagination.'

This show of shame is the contribution of the gates of hell to societal values. Even though it irritates the morally sensitive the corrupt mind sees it as an opportunity to pick new fashion trends that they may later spread among the ignorant masses and some members of the Church. This is the influence of the gates of hell.

xvi)They affect the Thinking of the Society and are Terribly Corrupt - The society at large is affected by the wrong signals the gates send out. They promote the flaunting of stolen wealth and make a thief a chief. The society is highly contaminated by the promotion of corrupt values from highest to the lowest. The society is built on the principles of survival of the fittest, and the smartest or the best thief gets the credit as merit is thrown overboard.

Their children are helped to pass their examinations and admissions are secured for them for large sums of money. Those that cannot beat them have now joined them, and this seems to have received the approval of the Nigerian society. Even some members of the Church, who are supposed to know better, are sometimes caught off guard as they approve the current practice with statements such as *"..Render... unto Caeser the things which are Caeser's.."* (Mt 22:21). It is a shame.

xvii) They are Noted for Promoting or Sponsoring Evil Cults

- The number of cults in Nigeria's university and polytechnic campuses have increased tremendously when compared to the few that existed in the 1970s and 1980s. Apart from the male dominated cults of those days, you now have purely female cult groups like the Jezebels on campus that bring down the reign of terror on the student populace.

Ordinarily, such groups should not survive the opposition of the strong arm of the law, except that there are powerful men and women in the society backing them as their patrons and matrons. Any attempt by the law enforcement agents to clamp down on them and arraign them for prosecution is usually frustrated as their hands suddenly become tied through pressures from above.

Surprisingly, some powerful parents are involved and they encourage their wards or are aware that their wards are involved in these cults and they do nothing about it. The recruitment drive is done secretly and powerfully too. They find easy recruits from lay-abouts who have nothing to do in the university. Some of these are students whose parents smuggled them into the university through fraudulent means. Of course, large sums of money actually exchanged hands in the wicked deal.

These students, unable to cope with the school system, jump from one night party to the other and inadvertently get initiated into the secret cult. By the time they realize the implications of what they are into, it would have become too dangerous to withdraw. So they become willing tools in the devils hands, and dare not tell anybody about it or else get killed. That is the reason why they keep to themselves, get high on drugs, talk less, become aggressive when slightly agitated, and remain willingly obedient to the ethics of the cult even to the point of death.

Their strong backers at times use them to fight their own 'private wars', which usually leaves many wounded and some dead. The law of 'an eye for an eye' that operates among cult members has left many dead,

and the lucky ones incarcerated for life. This situation is now dangerously affecting the fabric of the society so much so that every body including the government has come to agree that there is a need for divine intervention to deal with the situation.

xviii)They Promote Disguised Prostitution - The movers and shakers of the society largely encourage the prostitution you find in the nation today especially on   campus. Some of these girls are lured into this vice by inviting them to functions just to stand as chaperon or   ushers, but the allurement of riches and misplaced societal values find the weak ones among them in amorous relationships they did not bargain for.

The News Magazine of July 31st 2000 in the "QUOTES" Column corroborates this through the comments of the Special Adviser to the President on Women Affairs Chief (Mrs.) Titi Ajanaku on prostitution at home and abroad:

[2] "The ugly side of the matter is that some of our highly-placed men, holding public office cannot travel for conferences and seminars without these girls. The girls are not there to entertain them alone, but have fun with them."

The above statement is also confirmed by the report in the "News behind the news" (Nbtn) column of The Punch Group of Newspapers of April 6, 2001 on page 26. The story is titled 'The 40 wise girls':

[3] 'Several suggestively dressed girls acted as ushers at the southern governors conference. In all, they were 40 in number and were drawn from the University of Benin, College of Education, Benin, Federal Polytechnic, Auchi the Delta

State University, Abraka, and the Benin outreach campuses of Ladoke Akintola and Ondo State Universities. Over a thousand girls applied for the job but only the 40 passed the rigorous screening tests, which were said to be all encompassing.

For instance, during one of the screening sessions, Nbtn learnt that experts examined some 'exclusive' parts of the girls to detect possible 'crevices' where weapons could be concealed since they were to be allowed unfettered access to their excellencies. Many of the girls so pleased the governors that they went home with a lot of money which made their N3,000 allowance looked like a drop of rain.'

To show the seriousness of the matter at hand, the same newspaper on the same page carried a follow up story on the Southern Governor's Conference where the phobia of a governor's wife for the girls used as ushers was exposed. The paper gave in graphical details the anxiety expressed by a governor's wife and the desperate efforts she made to protect her beloved husband. Please find the interesting report quoted for your enjoyment. The paper said she was:

[*4] 'Not the type to take chances, she decided to follow her husband to the recently concluded conference….' And that she '…almost became her husbands appendage, because she followed him everywhere..'

Furthermore, she:

> ***5** '..had a running battle warding off rampaging young girls, who served as ushers, from snatching her husband on the dance floor. She insisted on dancing with him throughout, even when other governors took turns in engaging the damsels in fancy footwork.'

Can you blame her? The kingdom of God suffers violence and the violent ones take it by force. What further proof do we need of the rot that has pervaded the society? Only righteousness and truth can help the nation to return to a society that has the fear of God. So help us God.

xix)*They Promote Mediocrity* - The yardstick for appointment into public office is no longer probity, integrity, and merit but mediocrity. Wrong men are found occupying the right throne, and confusion has become   the order of the day, because fools or corrupt men are set in great dignity. Through their influence servants ride on horses, while princes walk as servants upon the earth as we see in Ecclesiastes Chapter 10:5-6.

> *"There is an evil which I have seen under the sun, as an error which proceedeth from the ruler: Folly is set in great dignity, and the rich sit in low place"*

xx) *Gates do not Release their Captives* - When gates operate it takes divine intervention to be delivered from their onslaught. This is because in the court of Satan the minimum prison sentence is life imprisonment, and the maximum sentence for offence committed is death. This is confirmed in the book of Isaiah 14:17: ***"…that openeth not the house of his prisoners?"***

Any body that suffers the misfortune of being locked up in Satan's prison house is in it for good. This is the reason some problems are generational or ancestral. Many families have suffered various degrees of protracted captivities in the hand of the devil. The pattern has always been the same down the line until God intervenes through His deliverance power because He is the one that ensures: ***"…. The opening of the prison to them that are bound."*** (Is. 61:1)

and

"..bringeth out those which are bound with chains…." (Ps. 68:6).

It is one thing to open the prison door, it is another thing entirely to be brought out of it intact, hale, and hearty. The door may be opened, and one may not have the strength to walk out because of poor condition of health. God ensures this is taken care of.

A good example of the wickedness of the devil is the encounter of King Hezekiah with the king of Assyria in II kings chapters 18:13-37 and 19: 1-37. Despite all entreaties, the enemy held on tightly to his captives until God intervened.

FIERY DART PRAYERS

1. Spirit of the living God, I break the power backing the gates of wickedness in the name of Jesus.

2. Let shame and disappointment be the portion of the wicked in Jesus name.

3. I cancel every covenant and desecrate the altar granting the wicked unusual power to oppress me.

4. I break the ranks of the wicked and send confusion into their midst in Jesus name.

5. Father, let every gathering of powers backing the wicked be scattered now.

6. Spirit of the living God, just like you frustrated the counsel of Ahitophel do the same to the counsel of these men in Jesus name.

7. O Lord! Frustrate their tokens and make their diviners mad in Jesus name.

8. Father, break the cheekbones of the enchanters that liberty may be granted to your people in Jesus name.

9. Let the adversaries of God be visited by thunder and lightening in Jesus name.

10. O Lord! let the confusion of the wicked be multiplied so that they would not know what to do in their calamity.

Chapter Five
THE MANIFESTATIONS OF SPIRITUAL GATES

'…..they afflict the just, they take a bribe, and they turn aside the poor in the gate from their right'. - Amos 5:12

Introduction

The evidence of the operation of spiritual gates is obvious in the lives of some families, and individuals. Realization and identification is usually made difficult as a result of people's attitude towards it, because many people think it cannot happen to them. Yet, forces of darkness bind many of them and satanic afflictions abound in many families, without any hope of deliverance.

The ignorance, demonstrated by men and the churches they belong to have compounded issues, and men have been forced to seek for help in wrong places, when faced with the realities on ground. As a result some have been abused, tormented, used, harassed, embarrassed and humiliated in the course of seeking for deliverance. Some even die prematurely during the process, leaving an impression of hopelessness to the members of the family, who are also facing the same problem in life.

Coupled with the weight of satanic affliction, the prayer lives of some have been battered so much so that the summary of their lives is that they alternate between mountain and valley experiences. What makes matters worse is that the things that used to be a walkover for them are now the subjects of prayers. Having wandered from pillar to post in search of help, ashes have settled upon their prayer altars and many unfulfilled dreams, and shattered hopes are all they have to show for all their efforts. They have fasted and prayed; yet nothing seems to have changed.

Their situation is presently a tale of woes and except something is done fast they may throw in the towel as frustration has set in. The book of Amos 5:12 tells us the secret behind this problem and these are the facts those that sit in the gate:

"...afflict the just, they take a bribe, and they turn aside the poor in the gate from their right".

They were supposed to guarantee the inalienable rights of the people but have turned their backs on them. They bring affliction upon the just, because they have been bribed to do so. Beyond the physical control, the spiritual rights of the people have been trampled upon by the powers that be and their lives, controlled from satanic altars. The supernatural powers they wield have been put into operation through sorcery to oppress the people and subject them to years of fruitlessness and hard labor.

Barriers of limited or conditional prosperity have been tied to some lives, so that whenever any member of that family overshoots that barrier by one dollar, he is suddenly cut down and dies. This is the reason why members of some families have not been able to outlive a certain age, successfully build houses, buy cars, succeed in business or even produce a graduate. The moment they exceed the limits that the gates have programmed into their lives they die, go insane, suddenly disappear, or an inexplicable misfortune happens to them.

It is however, clear from the Bible that it is our right to prosper, to be in health, and succeed in whatever we do. The book of III John 2 tells us:

"Beloved, I wish above all things that thou mayest prosper and be in health, even as thy soul prospereth".

This is very comforting and it shows that there is hope for the hopeless. This is reinforced by the book of Job 36:6 which tells us that he *"....giveth right to the poor".*

The right to live, rule, reign, prosper, be in health, be successful and fruitful in life. If this is so, why are we not prospering and entering into our inheritance in Christ? The book of Ezekiel 34:27 provides us with the answer:

"And the tree of the field shall yield her fruit, and the earth shall yield her increase, and they shall be safe in their land, and shall know that I am the Lord, when I have broken the bands of their yoke, and delivered them out of the hand of those that served themselves of them."

It is clear from the above verse that as long as the bands of their yoke are intact they can never be fruitful. The solution is in dealing with the bands of their yoke, and delivering them from the hand of the oppressor that is working against their success. The "***bands of their yoke***" are consequences of the operation of spiritual gates in their lives.

Many people have experienced limitations in life and have seen a regular sequence of such events passed down from generation to generation. They have a history of failure at the point of success and every attempt to go higher is thwarted by invisible barriers unknown to them. The gates have defined the limits of their success and how far they can go in life.

In order for them to break this barrier however, there must be divine intervention. Such men require not only deliverance but the revival of their prayer lives in order to maintain the checks on the forces of darkness operating in their lives. The first step towards victory however, is to identify and acknowledge the situation on ground, by seeking to know the operation, and manifestations of anomalies through a personal and realistic assessment of one's life.

A brother was busy playing the game of Table Tennis on his wedding day, while everybody was in church waiting for him. When his mother could no more contain her embarrassment she went in search of him, and after about thirty minutes of intensive searching, he found him in a compound playing Table Tennis. No matter how hard his mother tried to remind him of what was happening that day, he just could not remember that it was his wedding day. The enemy finished him completely, because the wedding was eventually cancelled.

A guide, which is by no means exhaustive, has been set out hereunder to help you identify if gates have been erected against your life and shut you out of your God-given inheritance. If we must enjoy the move of God in our land and experience the breakthrough Jesus promised us, we must confront these gates of wickedness.

i) **Consistent Inexplicable Limitation** - When a person repeatedly fails his examination without logical reasons; a marriage suddenly collapses or a person has repeated broken engagements; when a church is not growing; or a business fails in spite of all business prudence; where one has always been limited from getting a job, admission or promotion at the point of success even though qualified, they are all signs of gates at work. A good example is found in Genesis 5:25:

"And Methuselah lived an hundred and eighty and seven years, and begat Lamech."

The enemy so completely limited him that it took him one hundred and eighty seven years to have a son. This was a general problem in the land because of the ground God had cursed (Gen 3:17-19; Gen 5:29). The same limitation operated in the life of his son, who was one hundred and eighty two years before he had a son:

"And Lamech lived an hundred eighty and two years, and begat a son" (Gen. 5:28).

A similar limitation operated in the life of a brother who spent thirteen years studying to obtain a degree that would normally take four years. While limitations get you there very late, impossibility makes sure you never get there. This is the reason behind several engagements that never resulted in marriage. A sister received thirty-two proposals and had short-lived engagements that never ended in her walking down the aisle. If the partner did not die, he would have business failure that would lead to discouragement and eventual break-up of the relationship. The gates were at work, shutting men out of their inheritance.

ii) **Obvious Covering of Darkness Over a Land and its People** - Where this is in operation, the community experiences wickedness, immorality (prostitution, sodomy, etc), untimely death, poverty, high crime rate, murder and gross underdevelopment.

In situations like this, abnormalities become the norm. Men sit at home drinking alcohol, and laying about, while their women work themselves to the bone. There is a prevalence of idolatry, and operation of fetish powers in order to achieve peace at home and to prevent female 'hawks' from snatching already spoilt husbands. The society depends largely on all forms of sacrifice to keep hope alive, and by so doing goes deeper and deeper into bondage.

Those that are afflicted with this kind of bondage, usually belong to families that have suffered several generations of captivity, and deprivation. These families are usually restless, unfocussed, irrational, easily agitated and things never worked out for them. Their boys are destructive, crime prone and terribly violent, while their girls are wayward, and easily embrace prostitution, competing with adults in this business of death in spite of the AIDS scourge.

The communities in which this darkness dwells have more brothels and abortion clinics than schools and hospitals. Drugs of all sorts and alcohol are available to take them high and enable them perform any evil they choose with satanic vigor. Some use them initially to forget their sorrows, but as addiction sets in, they become easy recruits into the world of crime.

The satanic attack on the people limits the Church in such communities from entering into their inheritance, and as a result one begins to observe a high level of corruption, wickedness, inner wrangling, unhealthy competition, covetousness, love of money, infidelity, impurity and worldliness of the worst kind in the Church of God. Snatching of converts (not winning of souls), become a do or die affair, especially where big fish is involved.

As a result of this situation the churches are unable to settle down to achieve the building of the body of Christ. Their congregation consists of a recycled group of babies, year in year out that are unable to survive the least of temptations. They are therefore limited from enjoying God's promises for their lives. The gates are at work and there is a need to watch out.

iii) **Resistance to the Gospel** - Anywhere you see violent resistances to the gospel or the truth, gates are at work. The city gates of such communities have locked out the truth but have accommodated lies, and error. You will find shrines and covens more predominant as against a few struggling Churches. Witches and wizards boast and walk about doing their business in broad daylight. It is an abnormal thing in such places, not to have shrines or satanic altars in a home, because idolatry, and fetish powers are prevalent there. Such societies depend largely on all forms of sacrifice to keep hopes alive.

There was such a community that we went to minister to several years ago. It was an assignment that required dealing with the altars of affliction oppressing the people of the land. While the warfare lasted, I personally led a team of ministers to do a survey of the shrines and churches in the community. It was not a surprise to discover that the number of churches compared to shrines was ratio 1:10. Satanic shrines filled that land and the gospel was heavily hindered causing the people to suffer under the weight of affliction.

iv) **Deliberate Attempts to Pollute Godly Seeds** - This is much more pronounced among youths in the process of growth. The infiltration of the enemy into the church has brought in alien ideas, and norms of behavior. Our youths in their exuberance, under the guise of liberty of the spirit, have exceeded the normal bounds of decency, and unprintable and unimaginable vices are indulged in.

The society in general is being assaulted with satanic materials, video films, television programs, music, cartoons etc. Unsightly things are done publicly and righteous souls have their senses assaulted by all sorts of satanic clothes within and outside the church. Even the people of Sodom and Gomorrah would feel embarrassed at the level of depravity!

These are also the days when unimaginable ideas are proposed by Christians of long standing, such as pregnancy before marriage, trial marriages, sex before marriage, carousing or necking. Many of their children have gotten pregnant before marriage, and in some cases are married to stark unbelievers.

There is also a prevalence of disguised but coerced prostitution and sexual abuse inflicted on females in order for them to have breakthroughs in higher institutions, and business establishments. Many born again sisters, have been deliberately subjected to such evil attacks, by their occultist superiors who knew their stand as Christians yet insisted in having carnal knowledge of them before giving them pass marks to graduate.

While some struggle to keep their heads above the water, and put their hopes in God for deliverance, some have joined the Joneses, thus getting the godly seed polluted. When this is happening around you, watch out, the gates are after your inheritance!

Two sisters were under such intense pressure from their lecturer, for sexual relationships for many academic sessions. As a result of their refusal, they suffered various carry-overs of courses. In the final year when the reality of the possibility of not graduating dawned on them, both of them had a discussion, and resolved to allow the man have his way. At the end of the affair, the two of them got pregnant, and another round of trouble started in their lives.

In order to cover up the sin, both of them planned to trick their engaged suitors, into having carnal knowledge of them. One succeeded in forcing her partner into sin, while the other failed and was caught. Meanwhile, the one that succeeded rushed the brother into a quick marriage in order to cover the crime up.

Caught with an unwanted pregnancy, and no quick marriage in sight, the second sister had to confess - how in one night a lecturer slept with both of them and the follow up plan they both hatched. A calculation of the ages of both pregnancies corroborated the sister's story. It was only then that the other brother realized that he had been fooled into fathering a child that did not belong to him.

But our God must have a godly seed and nothing will hinder His plans to achieve this purpose. The word of God declares His strategy to achieve this in Malachi 3:15. He made two to become one in marriage. Why did He do so?

"That he might seek a godly seed"

It is therefore important to watch out the way you handle your marriage vows less you fall into the trap of the enemy to pollute your seed. The antidote is also in Malachi 2:15:

"Therefore take heed to your spirit and let none deal treacherously against the wife of his youth"

Take this warning my friend! Do not spend unnecessary time with a single sister during counseling or show unusual interest in her case. Avoid ungodly emotional attachment that draws you intimately to your so-called 'spiritual daughter' at the expense of your wife's feeling. Some 'spiritual fathers' have, during some unguided moments, been lured into having carnal knowledge of their 'spiritual daughters'. As a result they entered into the problem of fathering an unwanted ungodly seed. So be warned!

v) **Suffering in the Midst of Plenty** - Fear, intimidation, timidity, and complacency in the midst of poverty. It is as if the people are blind and cannot see their despicable spiritual situation. A few years of accumulated wealth in the country has been embezzled, squandered, or wasted by a few people. The consequent economic downturn, and constant hardship has led to frustration and some people have accepted this condition with equanimity.

The devil has fooled the people in believing a lie, and that is 'God will do it'. Instead of rising up to deal with the forces keeping them down in abject poverty, they live under this illusory consolation. Unknown to them, the Bible contradicts their confession making them to be liars as we see in Isaiah 44:23:

" Sing, O ye heavens for the Lord hath done it:.."

What further conviction do you need my friend? God has already done it, all that is left for you is to rise up and possess your possession. Ignorance and foolishness have however kept many going round in circles in an unending cycle of suffering and smiling.

The sad thing is that foreigners come in to steal and plunder, while the landowners dwell in the land as slaves. None is willing to pay the price for a breakthrough, because the gates have defined their limits. It is only the revival of God's word that can open the eyes of any one found in this condition. One needs to watch, pray, and rise up to confront these gates of limitation.

Many are unwilling to fast, pray, work, and trust the Lord for breakthroughs. They revel in philosophies that can produce no result but keep its proponents bound in abject poverty. You hear such statements like **'No condition is permanent'**, but they have neither done anything physical nor spiritual to change their conditions. My friend 'Pass me not O gentle Savior' is not a song you sing kneeling down. You must be on your feet, up and doing.

vi) **Repeated Afflictions, Sickness, and Tragedies** - Whether at national, community, family, or personal level when situations like these occur gates are at work. If, for example, you always find corrupt, wicked and ungodly men in various offices at all levels this is a national malady and tragedy!

Where something terrible always happens to you or somebody so dear to you, and always ends up causing irreparable damage or constitute a distraction, when you are about to write examination, go for an interview, execute a contract or catch up with a very important appointment, gates are at work in your life to hinder your progress.

vii) Reproach, Rejection, and Manipulation - When a person, family, people or nation comes under reproach, rejection, are despised and are being manipulated the gates are at work. The present reproach we face, as a nation is best imagined than experienced, when you fall into the hands of over zealous immigrations officers outside this country. Our reproach has been brought upon us on account of a collective curse, and the determination of Satan to destroy the image of this nation and its people. The reason for this is to limit this great nation from entering into its inheritance as a leader and an instrument in God's hands, to take the gospel to the nations and continents of the world.

On a personal level, if you find yourself in situations where everything initially points to a breakthrough, and the tide suddenly turns and you are told to keep coming only to be told at the last minute, 'We are sorry, try again next year' something is wrong somewhere. If a help, which seems assured suddenly becomes elusive, uncooperative, mischievous, manipulative, untruthful, in spite of the prior conviction that one had and you have noticed a sequence of such occurrences, then the gates have moved against you.

It also manifests in frequent termination of jobs, broken engagements almost at the point of marriage and deceptive relationships. It is common in such relationships for one party to find himself/herself unceremoniously jilted by the news that the fiancé/ fiancée has surreptitiously contracted a marriage out of state. The reproach this situation brings leads many weak ones to the precipice of insanity, especially when its regularity becomes too unbearable.

viii) **Barrenness, Un-fulfillment, and Relocation (Brain Drain)** - The nation's best brains have been frustrated and limited to the point of un-fulfillment. Major facilities have collapsed, basic amenities are lacking, and worse still we are living far below basic human conditions. Many are consequently forced to relocate, leaving the country in a more terrible state than it was.

On a personal level, where barrenness in marriage, business, or other venture is the case the problem is the same. It has resulted in unexpected divorces, relocation and in some cases getting involved in messy 'arrangee' marriages, which have worsened their situation. No matter what they do, some have remained unfulfilled in every aspect of their lives, and if you take a critical look at the problem, you would find the invisible hand of Satan trying to elicit frustration and introduce suicide into the life of the victim.

The first trick is to make the victim believe that relocation will solve the problem, forgetting that all the devil needs to do is to transfer their case file to the demons in charge of the place they are relocating to in order to continue the affliction. Many people have fallen into this trap, and have ended up a nervous wreck, who has to work round the clock at menial jobs to survive. The gates have achieved their purpose in that life.

Conclusion

The first step towards victory as stated earlier on is to acknowledge the situation on ground, through a personal and realistic assessment of one's life and stop pretending. Behaving as if it does not exist does not help matters. It is obvious to all that they are bound, yet they carry on as if nothing is happening. This is the reason for the number of casualties being recorded in our various Churches, as many die before their time because they fail to seek for help.

There is a need for the saints to arise in the place of prayers. We must go to the mountaintop where we must cry our hearts out until we receive deliverance. We must begin to walk in holiness in order to possess our possessions. We must endeavor to fly high as the way of the eagle is in the sky. It is time to say no to sorrow, tears, and bloodshed. Stand up to the oppressor, whip him, and get the victory in Christ through prayers. The Church of Christ must be built, and the gates of hell shall not prevail against it.

FIERY DART PRAYERS

1.   I come against the arrowhead of evil stationed to monitor my life and forbid them from to manifesting in my life in the name of Jesus.

2.   In the name of Jesus, I dismantle the arrowhead of evil setup in my lineage to destroy me.

3.   I come against satanic consortium of evil gathered together to upstage me in life in Jesus name.

4.   In the name of Jesus, I command every manifestation of satanic gates to cease in my life.

5.   I decree that loss of memory become the portion of sorcerers that are working against my success in life.

6.   I speak to the stars in their courses that they should begin to fight against every Sisera in my life.

7.   Just as the morning introduces the day, let the sun of glory introduce my glory in God.

8.   Every satanic brief of judgment collected against me is today visited with the Holy Ghost fire.

9.   I reject every satanic agreement binding my family to disaster, destruction, and disappointments.

10.   I open the door of my life to prosperity, success, health, and abundance in Jesus name.

Chapter Six
WARFARE STRATEGIES

"...Behold I lay in Zion for a foundation a stone, a tried stone, a precious corner stone, a sure foundation.." - *Isaiah 28:16*

Attitude Required for Spiritual Warfare

In order to deal with the kingdom of darkness, we require the right approach in line with that of a follower of Christ. A restless or rash person cannot survive in spiritual warfare. An impulsive, person who is quick to react will regret ever going into warfare with the wrong approach that is if he ever survives to tell the story. The book of Isaiah chapter 41 verse 1, reveals to us the right approach to spiritual warfare:

"Keep silence before me, O islands; and let the people renew their strength: let them come near; then let them speak: let us come near together to judgment".

This verse of scripture clearly gives us a step-by-step strategy to adopt for victory in prayer warfare and is set out as follows:

i)   *"Keep silence before me", - Watching in Prayer, Key to Revelation*. Revelation is a key issue in spiritual warfare and when dealing with spiritual gates it cannot be over emphasized. Having recognized the existence of the problems, it is important to know the source, and legal reason for their existence. This key will enable the intercessor to have specific instructions from the headquarters as to what to do in handling specific cases of affliction.

It is very important to mention that prayer basically must be Holy Ghost inspired. Thus, when faced with the task of dealing with the forces of darkness wisdom demands that a spiritual man must keep silent in order to receive clear directives from the spirit of God. Inspiration flows better when this is observed. The book of II Chronicles 20:1-4, 13-19 gives us an example of waiting in silence before him.

ii) *"O Islands" is a Snare, Corporate Anointing Required* - In the sight of God and men, Islands are those who believe they know it all and so they neither submit to direction, nor participate in team work. They are loners who believe so much in themselves to the point of deception, yet the gospel according to Saint Luke in Chapter 10 verse 1 tells us that the Lord Jesus:

"...sent them two and two before his face into every city and place, whither he himself would come."

Whether we like it or not spiritual warfare is better handled on corporate level. That is why the Bible says in II Corinthians 10:4:

"For the weapons of our warfare are not carnal...".

Note that the Bible says:

"our warfare" not *"my warfare"*.

According to scriptures also one shall chase a thousand and two shall chase ten thousand (Dt. 32:30). The secret of victory is to submit to God's divine strategy in order to walk in the glorious liberty of God's victory.

iii) *"Let the people renew their strength"*, *Aggressive Prayer and Fasting* - The Lord Jesus gave us an idea of what this kind of battle requires in the gospel of Mark 9:29:

"This kind can come forth by nothing, but by prayer and fasting."

Warfare requires renewed strength because every battle fought saps a man's strength. This is also true of our daily service to humanity, thus the strength of yesterday cannot be used to fight today's battle.

Every soldier must renew his strength. The Biblical way a spiritual soldier renews his strength is mentioned in Isaiah 40:31:

"But they that wait upon the Lord shall renew their strength…".

This is simply waiting upon the Lord in fasting, prayers, word meditation, and in-depth study of the word of God. Whatever increased energy level acquired during this period, will be useful to confront the gates of the enemy:

"And it shall be said in that day, Lo, this is our God; we have waited for him, and he will save us: this is the Lord; we have waited for him, we will be glad and rejoice in his salvation" (Is 25:9).

iv) *"Let them come near"*, - *Having a Vibrant Prayer Altar* - The next step after fulfilling the first three is to draw near to God and this in other words, is submitting to God. Some pray to God but they are far from him. The Bible reveals that during the trial of Jesus *"..Peter followed him afar off.."* (Mat. 26:58). I believe this is the problem of some of us. We pray afar off. Why is this so? Un-repented sin e.g. malice, bitterness, un-forgiveness, backbiting, and other forms of sin are the things that keep us away from God. Repentance and holy living draw you closer to God. It is when you get close to God that you can make your desires known to him. The counsel of James 4:7 becomes relevant here:

"Submit yourself therefore to God. Resist the devil, and he will flee from you."

It is through submission or surrendering of self in all things that you can have victory in spiritual warfare.

v) "Then let them speak", - Prophetic Utterance and Action – When the pathway to prayer has been cleared through repentant communion with God, speaking to Him your desires easily follows. This is the point where you resist the devil and make prophetic declarations over your life or situation. Do not speak except you are sure you are spiritually near to Him and then the following steps should be helpful in approaching Him:

a) "Enter into his gates with thanksgiving" (Ps 100:4). The key that opens the gate is thanksgiving and the one that opens his court is praise. You need to symbolically enter into his gates with praise. This is very necessary in spiritual warfare: *"And at midnight Paul and Silas prayed, and sang praises unto God: and the prisoners heard them.*

And suddenly there was a great earthquake, so that the foundations of the prison were shaken: and immediately all the doors were opened, and every one's bands were loosed." (Acts. 16:25-26).

b) "Open ye the gates", (Is 26:2). The gate must be opened in order that the righteous nation, which 'keepeth' the truth, may enter in. Without it opening you cannot make progress spiritually and physically. Therefore you must command the gates to be opened:

Open thy doors, O Lebanon, that the fire may devour thy cedars" (Zech. 11:1).

c) *"Lift up your heads, o ye gates"* (Ps 24:7). You must demand that this scripture should be fulfilled. The gates must be lifted up for the Lord to come in and take possession his church. This is the battle of words, and the words must be released to effect the changes required. You must be prophetic and daring as the Holy Spirit leads you in the battle.

d) *Ask:* This is simply making your request known to God in the simplest way possible. Prayer is not supposed to be a complicated art, but men have introduced complication into this God-given way of relating with Him. In spite of this however, God continues to declare:

"Ask of me, and I shall give thee the heathen for thine inheritance, and the uttermost parts of the earth for thy possession" (Ps 2:8).

This counsel is necessary when dealing with gates, because spiritual gates lock men out of their inheritance and dispossess them of their blessings in life. By asking you are making a demand to possess the heathen in order for you to recover all he has stolen from you. Then you need to go ahead and: "***...break them with a rod of iron; thou shalt dash them in pieces like a potter's vessel***" (Ps 2:9)

vi) ***"Let us do judgment" By Possessing the Gates of the Enemy*** – It is at this stage that full-scale spiritual warfare is entered into. Anything done irrationally before this time may attract grave consequences. The **'us'** here is you and the Holy Spirit in the place of prayer. This we see clearly highlighted in Romans 8:26. The Holy Spirit helps our infirmities. More explicitly expressed is the reference in Ps 82:1:

"***God standeth in the congregation of the mighty; he judgeth among the gods***".

This has been made possible only by the existence of a deep prayer relationship with Him. Executing judgment consists of:

a) ***Possessing the Gates of your Enemies (G****en 22:17). You must prayerfully take possession and prophetically make declarations to this effect.

b) ***Breaking the Gates*** (107:16*)* - The gates of brass and bars of iron that have shut you out of your inheritance must be aggressively addressed. Command every one of these to be broken to pieces and speak to them to be opened to breakthrough including the evangelization of your community.

c) *Making the Gates of the Enemy Desolate* (Lam 1:4). The strategy of God in battle is to have outright victory and failure to accomplish this may result in your own lamentation as it happened in Lamentation chapter 1 verse 4:"*....all her gates are desolate: her priests sigh, her virgins are afflicted, and she is in bitterness*"

So before the enemy strikes, hit him so hard that he will never recover from the desolation:

"*For thou hast made of a city an heap; of a defenced city a ruin: a palace of strangers to be no city; it shall never be built.*" (Is 25:2)

d) *Destroying the Gates* (Is 24:12) - While dealing with the gates, ensure that they, and their

"*...city* (are) *left* (in) *desolation, and the gate is smitten with destruction*".

e) *Sinking the Gates* (Lam 2:9) - Finally, take authority over the gates, and sink them, making the place vulnerable for constant assault. The man of God Moses had to release a word like this in Numbers 16:30:

"*But if the Lord make a new thing, and the earth open her mouth, and swallow them up, with all that appertain unto them, and they go down quick into the pit; then ye shall understand that these men have provoked the Lord*"

The Bible declares what happened thereafter in verses 31 and 32:

" And it came to pass, as he had made an end of speaking all these words, that the ground clave asunder that was under them: And the earth opened her mouth, and swallowed them up...".

These strategies will help you to sort out the bottlenecks experienced through unanswered prayers. Meditate on the verses quoted and observe the principle; the Lord will surprise you as you do so.

FIERY DART PRAYERS

1. Open thy doors, O ye wicked, that the fire may devour thy gates in Jesus name.

2. O Lord, according to your word in Psalm 2:8 I ask for the heathen for my inheritance in Jesus name.

3. O Lord, according to your word in Psalm 2:9 I take possession of the heathen today in Jesus name.

4. I break the heathen operating in my life with a rod of iron and dash them in pieces like a potter's vessel.

5. Spirit of the living God, I break the gates of the enemy today in Jesus name.

6. I sink the gates of the enemy and visit her and her virgins with affliction in Jesus name.

7.   I possess the gates of the enemy in Jesus name.

8.   I destroy the gates with the hammer of the word of God.

9.   In the name of Jesus, let every gate standing between me, and my inheritance sink now.

10.   I scatter the powers working against me.

Chapter Seven
HOW TO DEAL
WITH SPIRITUAL GATES

"In that day shall the Lord of hosts be for a crown of glory, and for a diadem of beauty, unto the residue of his people. And for a spirit of judgment to him that sitteth in judgment, and for strength to them that turn the battle to the gate." - Isaiah 28:16

Introduction

Dealing with the gates of the enemy requires some level of insight into spiritual warfare. This insight will enable one to develop effective strategies to handle the forces of darkness. In dealing with the gates the series of strategies identified are picked from the book of Isaiah 28 verses 16-21. The basic strategies are in themselves also weapons one should apply when dealing with the gates. The knowledge of these will assist the intercessor to hit at the foundation of evil gates in a person's life.

Strategies/Weapons

There are various weapons of war mentioned in the Bible. These are the word of God as a hammer, fire and sword, the name and blood of Jesus, the east wind, and the fire of the Holy Spirit etc. In addition to all these, other biblically relevant weapons that can be used against forces of darkness are itemized.

These weapons can be effectively utilized in worded prayers, that is, quoting copiously relevant portions of the Bible. One must be well grounded in the word of God to effectively fight at this level of warfare. The weapons are listed below:

i)   *Precious Corner Stone:* The book of Isaiah Chapter 28   verse 16 states:

   ".... Behold I lay in Zion for a foundation a stone, a tried stone, a precious corner stone, a sure foundation...".

   This is a reference to the Lord Jesus Christ, who was a rejected stone that became the head of the corner. This stone is a sure foundation and as you pray you must stand on this verse as your foundation for the battle. The stone is both a foundation (weapon of defense) and stone of assault (weapon of offence).

   Command the stone to sink into the forehead of the enemy and break its feet into pieces. There are two examples of this in the scriptures:

"And David put his hand in his bag, and took thence a stone and slang it, and smote the Philistine in his forehead, that the stone sunk into his forehead..."
(I Sam 17:49)

Also in the book of Daniel chapter 2 verse 34:

"Thou sawest till that a stone was cut out without hands, which smote the image upon his feet that were of iron and clay, and brake them to pieces."

ii) Judgment Laid to the Line: In verse 17 we see the words *"Judgment also will I lay to the line..."* Anytime you see the word 'line' or 'lines' the way it is used here, it speaks of the measuring line of your portion of inheritance as we see revealed in Psalm 16 verse 6:

"The lines are fallen unto me in pleasant places; yea, I have a goodly heritage" (My bible margin reads *'I have beautiful possessions'*).

The judgment here is a reference to the intervention of the just God in restoring all your stolen possessions or inheritance. Pray that God should lay judgment to the line and restore to you your stolen possessions in Jesus name. (Ref: John 10:10).

iii) Righteousness to the Plummet: *V*erse 17 continues with the following words

".... and righteousness to the plummet..."

We see here a continuation of the measuring line. While justice is laid to the line, righteousness is the instrument or plummet (or plumb-line) of ensuring the straightness of the line of your inheritance. The Amplified translation reads:

"I will make justice the line, and righteousness the plummet…",

While the New American Standard version renders it thus:

"And I will make justice the measuring line, and righteousness the level…."

In Zech 1:18-21 we see how the horns or gates scattered Judah, so that no man did lift up his head, but the corporate anointing of four carpenters (intercessors) delivered them from the horns (gates). You can prayerfully insist that you must rise above the limitation or *"..the level.."* the gates have placed upon you in Jesus name.

iv) ***Invoke the Ministry of the Hailstones:*** Hailstones are pellets of ice that fall from the clouds. God has also used this against the gates of hell "*…. and the hail shall sweep away the refuge of lies…"* (v17).

Even though lies have been their refuge the ministry of hailstones will sweep them away from our land. This weapon was effectively utilized in the book of Joshua Chapter 10 verse 11:

"And it came to pass, as they fled from before Israel and were in the going down to Beth-horon, that the Lord cast down great stones from heaven upon them unto Azekah, and they died: they were more which died with hailstones than they whom the children of Israel slew with the sword."

v) ***Waters Overflowing the Hiding Place:*** The water of God's word must be released to overflow the hiding place of the enemy. God did this to Pharaoh and his host in Exodus 14:28-29:

"And the waters returned, and covered the chariots, and the horsemen, and all the host of Pharaoh that came into the sea after them; there remained not so much as one of them...and Israel saw the Egyptians dead upon the sea shore"

vi) ***Annul the covenant with:*** It is important at this stage to cancel all evil covenants with death because Isaiah 7 verse 7 states that:

"..It shall not stand, neither shall it come to pass."

Why will it not come to pass? It is because God is with us. (Is 8:9-10)

vii) ***Cancel Agreement with Hell:*** When men are in agreement with hell, they fear nobody. Whether one believes it or not this agreement is binding on all the people living in that territory. Ignorance is no excuse in spiritual matters. No matter what the people try to do all hell will break loose upon them because of the agreement:

"Can two walk together, except they be agreed?" (Amos 3:3)

Break every evil agreement with failure, poverty, barrenness, and slow progress. Do not explain it away by saying **"It is common in my family"**. Rise up and cancel this ancient agreement and begin to enjoy the covenant heaven has entered into on your behalf through our Lord Jesus Christ.

viii)Release the overflowing scourge: The overflowing scourge in this respect is ceaseless prayers and fasting. The Bible says concerning the righteous that:

"Thou shalt be hid from the scourge of the tongue..." (Job 5:21).

We thank God that this provision does not cover the wicked, so we can release this overflowing scourge day and night. Let it be that from the time you commence these prayers it shall overtake them every morning, every day and night.

"From the time that it goeth forth it shall take" them, *"..morning by morning shall it pass over, by day and by night: and it shall be a vexation* (sheer terror) *only to understand the report* (message)" (Is 28:18-19).

ix) Make their bed shorter and their covering narrower:
-(Is 28:20). This is simply hitting hard at the base of
their peace and comfort. When a man's:

"***...bed is shorter than that a man can stretch
himself on it: and covering narrower than that he
can wrap himself in it***" he has double portion of
affliction.

He has lost his rest and peace, and will die very soon
of cold. This is a disaster you must bring upon the
enemy.

x) Let God Arise: It is important to firmly ask the
Lord to arise in order for the enemy to be scattered
in different directions. In the book of the Prophets:
Isaiah 28 verse 21 we see such an act of God:

"***For the Lord shall rise up as in mount Perazim,..***"

Why should He rise up? He would rise up, so that
He can make Himself known to all His enemies. The
concluding verse confirms this. It states that God
should arise so that:

"***...he may do his work, his strange work; and
bring to pass his act, his strange act***"

He will do His strange work and bring to pass his
strange act over your lives in Jesus name; only if you
can pray.

FIERY DART PRAYERS

1. I rise above the limitation the gates have placed upon my life in the name of Jesus because justice is the measuring line of my inheritance

2. O Lord let righteousness be the level of my rising in life in Jesus name.

3. I command the precious corner stone of victory to and break the feet of the enemy into pieces in Jesus name.

4. I command the precious corner stone of victory to sink into the forehead of the enemy in Jesus name.

5. Father, in the name of Jesus lay judgment to the line and restore to me all my stolen possessions.

6. I invoke the ministry of hailstones to scatter the assembly of evil men against my promotion.

7. O Lord, I ask that you give me the heathen for my inheritance, and the uttermost parts of the earth for my possession according to your word in Psalm 2:8

8. O Lord, let the hail sweep away the refuge of lies raised against my life.

9. In the name of Jesus I annul every covenant with death.

10 Every agreement with hell against me shall not stand neither shall it come to pass.

Chapter Eight
SMASHING THE GATES

"And I say unto you that thou art Peter, and upon this rock I will build my church and the gates of hell shall not prevail against it." - *Mathew 16:18*

The Call to Battle

The truth many of us have failed to realize is that, every commitment made to Jesus in the place of receiving him as Lord and Savior is recruitment into the army of Christ. This army is the church that Jesus is building for the last day's battle against the forces of darkness. This Church is the one He boasted about in the gospel of Mathew chapter 16 verse 18:

"I will build my church and the gates of hell shall not prevail against it"

If this is so, every child of God must be prepared for battle. In other words it is a call for battle. A soldier should always be ready for service. He can be called upon on a very short notice to defend his nation, and he has no choice but to heed the call. The same applies to a spiritual soldier. He must be willing to heed the counsel of Apostle Paul in 2 Tim 2:3-4, which reads thus:

"Thou therefore endure hardness, as a good soldier of Jesus Christ.

No man that warreth entangleth himself with the affairs of this life; that he may please him who hath chosen him to be a soldier".

Once again, whether a soldier likes it or not, the moment he enlists into the army, he must be prepared for war. A person who is a soldier and feels otherwise is either ignorant or mischievous. His life also must reflect the discipline of the military. The first thing he loses is his liberty. Everything he does from then on must be ordered from above. The **"bloody civilian"** aspect of him must be thoroughly purged under pressure through rigorous military exercises. He must obey his commander, and superior officers or else he will run into trouble.

The safety of a soldier's life in any battle is guaranteed, if only he can submit to military authority. The commander has the ability to organize battle strategies, and read the course or direction a battle engaged in is headed. Therefore, disobedience to his instructions may portend serious danger to a recalcitrant soldier. This is all the more true also in spiritual warfare, because the war is not against flesh and blood. Obedience to the words of our commander in chief, the Lord Jesus Christ is our guarantee to safety.

All that is expected of an earthly soldier is equally expected of a spiritual soldier. If the **"bloody civilian"** attitude is decried in the secular, it is also not permitted in the spiritual army. The verse 4 of 2 Timothy Chapter 2 is clear in this respect:

"No man that warreth entangleth himself with the affairs of this life".

A good soldier stays in the barracks to receive military training. He is not allowed to break barracks rules. Training programs may however sometimes take him to jungles, thick forests, open fields, rivers, and mountainous or hilly paths in order to learn how to fight on various terrains. Most of these trainings are done very early in the morning, and some in the dead of the night to sharpen skills, and handling of nocturnal enemies.

A soldier must be trained on the use of various light and heavy artillery. These include short and long-range firearms and ammunition. In a nutshell, he must be trained in the use of conventional and unconventional weapons. Included in the training are early morning road walks for several kilometers for building up stamina. The sum of it all is that a good soldier must endure hardness.

Therefore in order to be effectively useful to smash the gates of the enemy the spiritual soldier must also stay in the 'spiritual barracks' (church and fellowship) to receive spiritual warfare training. He is not allowed to break 'spiritual barracks' (church and fellowship) rules. He must receive training at various Camp Meetings, Conferences, Seminars, Programs, and Bible Colleges etc. Just as these are mandatory for the secular soldier, so it is for the spiritual soldier.

To be a result-oriented soldier, learn to fight on all terrain, discourage the defensive, and generally ineffective rather-too-late warfare pattern, and be on the offensive. The laissez faire attitude towards the devil or the belief that if I do not trouble the devil, he will not bother me cannot help you in the day of trouble. Whether you do not talk about him in order not to glorify him or stir him up or not he is waiting for a time to strike. Why allow him to strike first? Adopt a pre-emptive strike strategy and you will walk in victory all the time.

It Is Time To Fight

The truth brother is that you must fight. Our Lord and Master have already made the call to battle. The battle of the last days is upon us. So that the: **'...kingdoms of this world** (may) **become the kingdoms of our Lord and of his Christ'**. (Rev 11:15)

Do not sit on the fence. It is either you fight or perish. In order to fight effectively however, you must continue to make use of the war strategies that your have learnt in order to acquire skills with which to fight. Practice makes perfect. Therefore, wake up early in the morning to do prayer warfare. Fight the good fight of faith even into the dead of the night to sharpen your skills in the handling of nocturnal enemy activities. Build up spiritual stamina through long periods of prayer and fasting. Give time to the study of the word (sword of the spirit) and meditation, which is the equivalent of light and heavy weapon training in the army.

As mentioned earlier the statement of the Lord Jesus in the gospel of Mathew chapter 16 verse 18 is a vicarious commitment to war. This is a declaration of war and the devil does not take statements like this for granted. You have no choice in the matter. To remain with him you must ensure that your weapons of war are intact.

If the church is a corpse, or is in the congregation of the dead, how can it successfully match the words of Jesus with action? How can it wage war against the gates of hell? Notice that the gates are not immobile so it is either you move against them or they move against you. I want you to understand that when Jesus said that: " *...the gates of hell shall not prevail against it".*

He was just reiterating the fact that you must advance against the gate. Do not wait for the gate to take the initiative. Go and deal with the gate. Confront the issues of your life and address them with violence. Let the enemy have no breathing space. Every seeming obstacle in our lives that has continued to terrify us is a gate and must be smashed open, but for you to do so you must believe that victory is yours, and that you can do it. Make up your mind to confront the gates of the enemy, which has put you under the siege of fear for many generations and smash them to pieces. All you need to do is to stand up and declare war against them. You will be surprised at what the Lord will do for you by defeating your enemy.

Overcome Fear

Fear is the outrider of failure and defeat. The Bible assures us in Isaiah 41:10:

"Fear thou not: for I am with thee: be not dismayed: for I am thy God: I will strengthen thee: yea, I will help thee: yea, I will uphold thee with the right hand of my righteousness."

All you need to do is to trust him to help you in times like this. The devil enjoys intimidation and is a master strategist in the use of psychological warfare. Many have been cowed by just empty threats, only to discover to their chagrin many years later that the enemy has a glass jaw. If they had been willing, and obedient, all they needed to have done was to have planted an upper cut on the enemy's jaws, but fear kept them from doing it, and they remained the worse for it.

Stand with God in judgment

In these last days the Lord is moving the church forward in the battle against the gates of hell. It is clear in the scriptures that: *"**God standeth in the congregation of the mighty: he judgeth among the gods.**"* (Ps 82:1)

Why? This is proof of God's approval of our exploits in prayer. God standing in the congregation of the mighty is a confirmation of the declaration of war against Satan. Who are the mighty? The mighty are those that have been redeemed, and given the power to be called the sons of God. We become mighty by entering into a covenant relationship with him. We take his strength and he takes our weakness upon himself, thus the Bible declares in I John 4:4 that: *"....**greater is he that is in you, than he that is in the world**"*.

The will of God is that we should manifest both His militant as well as his loving nature. This balance must be constantly demonstrated. The Lord declares that a combination of Himself, and us would make for signs and wonders: *"**Behold, I and the children whom the Lord hath given me are for signs and for wonders in Israel from the Lord of hosts, which dwelleth in mount Zion.**"* (Is. 8:18).

This cannot happen except a man abides in Him, and in His presence. The build up of fellowship and trust results in being equipped for battle. The word of God warns us in the gospel of Luke chapter 11 verses 21 to 22 that, when:

*"....**a strong man armed keepeth his palace, his goods are in peace:**"*

But when a stronger than he shall come upon him, and overcome him, he taketh from him all his armour wherein he trusted; and divideth his spoils."

This cannot be achieved except a man submits to Him. He will glorify Himself through us only if we allow Him to do so. Why will he judge among the gods? It is because the Lord Jesus said:

"All power is given unto me in heaven and in earth." (Mt. 28:18)

And that power and glory had been given to the children of God:*"And the glory which thou gavest me I have given them:.."* (John 17:23)

As we pray, and issue decrees, we are exercising dominion through Him. He ministers to us and through us. He is with us in every battle and willing to grant us victory as we move out in faith. When men gather together to pray he is there. That is the gathering of gods - those that have been redeemed. How do we know that the gathering is of the redeemed? Let us turn to John 10:34-35:

"Jesus answered them is it not written in your law, I said ye are gods. If he called them gods unto whom the word of God came and the scripture cannot be broken."

The word of God has come to you, and is still coming, to as

many as will receive Him and the moment they do they shall become the sons of God. In addition, they will receive power, and as the Holy Spirit fills them they receive fire. The provision of power and fire is for them to do exploits. The exploits in turn are to convert the kingdoms of this world unto the kingdoms of our Lord:

"And the seventh angel sounded and there were great voices in heaven saying the kingdoms of this world are become the kingdoms of our Lord and of his Christ and he shall reign for ever and ever". (Rev 11:15)

God has put a lot of premium on man. He desires a man to work with especially in the place of prayer. The prayer life of a man affects the happenings in heaven and on earth. This becomes so salient when you realize that a clarion call came from heaven asking the intercessors to bless the Lord so that God can bless them out of Zion:

"Behold, bless ye the Lord, all ye servants of the Lord, which by night stand in the house of the Lord. Lift up your hands in the sanctuary, and bless the Lord. The Lord that made heaven and earth bless the out of Zion." (Ps134:1-3)

"Ye that stand in the house of the Lord, in the courts of the house of our God, Praise the Lord; for the Lord is good: sing praises unto his name; for it is pleasant." (Ps. 135:2-3).

These are men that stand with the Lord by night in prayer; know the importance of such prayers, and also know the danger of not doing so. Since witches and wizards operate mostly at night these men lose their sleep in order to spike their activities and ensure the progress of God's work as well as the peace of the people on the earth, because it is

".... while men slept, his enemy came and sowed tares among the wheat, and went his way.' (Mt 13:25).

These men walk so closely with God that they are called saviors in the book of Obadiah verse 21:

"And saviours shall come up on mount Zion to judge the mount of Esau: and the kingdom shall be the Lord's."

They are also deliverers who have come to understand that for every mountain of Zion there is a mount of Esau to contend with. Their duty is to judge the mountain of Esau in order for the kingdom to be the Lord's. These are men who operate on kingdom principles. They are not fighting to build empires for themselves. Their hearts are totally knit with that of God that they feel pain when the kingdom goals are not achieved. This is the reason why God declared in Ps 149:4-9 that the Lord takes pleasure in the victory of His people. He insists on praise and the word (sword) as instruments to use:

"To execute vengeance upon the heathen, and punishments upon the people; To bind their kings with chains, and their nobles with fetters of iron;

To execute upon them the judgment written: this honour have all his saints..." (Ps 149:7-9)

Every believer who is willing to pay the price in the place of prayer and fasting has this honor of executing vengeance upon the heathen, punishment upon the people, binding the kings with chains, and the nobles with fetters.

One must however, guard against carelessness and overconfidence, which enabled the enemy to strike at the lives of the men who stood with God in Ps 82:1. Prayer time and personal fellowship with God began to diminish. Attraction for the things of the world began to fill the vacuum created. Then what used to arouse righteous indignation started receiving unrighteous recognition and standing ovation. Even though they continued to pray, their prayers became stereotyped, routine (the head praying without the heart), so they began to bring forth wrong judgments, and accept the persons of the wicked.

The purpose for which they were called - the fatherless, poor, needy, and afflicted was abandoned and when God had waited too long for them to repent, He cried out:

"How long will ye judge unjustly and accept the persons of the wicked........." (Ps. 82:2).

The problem of these backsliders is described in the scripture as ignorance and lack of understanding:

"They know not, neither will they understand; they walk on in darkness..." (Ps 82:5).

The sad thing here is that their prayerless lives affected both man, and the rest of creation. Their acceptance of wicked men gave a leeway to evil in the land, and disrupted even the foundations of the earth to the point that they went out of course: ***"..all the foundations of the earth are out of course"*** (Ps 82:5).

This problem facilitated the judgment of God upon the heathen who caused more problems for the people of God by remaining at ease in spite of the crisis at hand. Hence, in the book of Zechariah Chapter 1 verse 15 God stated his displeasure in the following words:

"...I am very sore displeased with the heathen that are at ease: for I was but a little displeased, and they helped forward the afflictions" .

Consequently, they continued to have fellowship with darkness. Even though a great light had been revealed, in their terrible condition they could not perceive it and so they remained in darkness. God became angry and sent forth His judgment, in an earthquake, which shook the foundations of the earth. The result of sin is always destruction and death; and people perish, because of lack of knowledge.

God is looking for a man

Men that were supposed to sustain the cause of God teamed up with evil and things went out of hand. This act of treason affected the whole of creation - the people and the earth. They allowed darkness to continue unabated, because they chose the path of rebellion and did not follow the injunction of the

Lord in spreading the light. They promoted evil men by recommending evil men to take over the portion of saints.

The Holy Spirit was no more a guide but a backbencher in their ministry because they found **"another key"** for success. As a result of the morbid condition of their hearts, the deceived, hypocrites, ungodly men, and women found comfortable pews in their Churches. The doctrines of God have gone through several refinements to suit the whims and caprices of the prime worshippers who rule the church from the altar of Mammon rather than the altar of God. What used to call for several days of strong crying between the porch, and altar had now become trivialized by a round table discussion of the board members. The foundation laid for light through prayer had been allowed to go: "... ***out of course.***" (Ps 82:5).

Man was placed in dominion to rule the world. The world can truly be ruled on our knees but we have let dominion slip through our hands through democratic processes. Democracy is good but God is not a democrat. God rules from the heavens and has given us power to do exploits. Except we see through the eyes of God we may be tempted to adopt a laissez faire attitude towards the devil. The devil does not believe in dialogue. The only language he understands is force.

"And from the days of John the Baptist until now the kingdom of heaven suffereth violence and the violent take it by force". (Mt 11:12)

I love the way the New International Version (NIV) translation puts it

"...*the kingdom of God has been forcefully advancing, and forceful men lay hold of it..*".

This brings to mind the story of a brother who was intimidated by six witches who through sorcery took dominion of the house in which he lived. The witches wanted total control and freedom to operate, and so waited for the right time to strike.

In the early hours of one morning as the brother retuned from vigil singing, he entered through the back door of his house, and saw the unexpected. Of the eight rooms in that house, six had their doors ajar and the occupants had their legs planted on the wall. His heart failed him instantly, because he understood the meaning of their actions. These were witches in manifestation. Within a matter of minutes, he packed all the light items of his property, and made rapid dialogue with his legs. He ran away and the witches succeeded in their assignment.

Another brother was subjected to the same treatment. This one did not even wait to pack anything. Not even a pin. He was visibly shaken and having no strength within him anymore he cried out, **"God forbid that a prophet should die outside Jerusalem"** and he ran out of that house like a kid pursued by a hungry lion.

There was another brother who took the battle to the gate. He was willing to smash the gates of the enemy by force. The moment he saw them, he gave them the riot act. "So you are witches. You are all in trouble in this house", he stated. He immediately declared war on them with a seven-day prayer and fasting retreat. By the time he got to the third day, violent reactions broke out from the camp of the enemy. The witches who were agitated and deeply affected by the heat of the operations in the heavenly places reported the brother to the landlord who happened to be the head of the community.

At a meeting called to settle the matter, the accusation raised against the brother was that he was praying too much. The arbitrator told them he could not do anything about that, but advised them to go and pray in return, as he would not adjudge praying as a sin. He then dismissed them.

This spiritual warfare that followed drew them into spiritual face-to-face combat that sent the six women packing one by one out of that house. The brother applied strategic level warfare by first breaking their spiritual backbone, unseat them from the realm of the spirit, and thereby cause their physical evacuations to be effected. A child of God who knew his God, and was strong and could do exploits terminated the siege of witches over the house.

The three kinds of men mentioned above are also identified in Gideon's army of 32,000 men. When the call was made, they heeded the call in the flesh, but when God began to apply qualifying measures the number reduced. The parameter of fear eliminated 22,000 men from the crowd and 10,000 men were left. When the parameter of lapping water like dogs was used the 10,000 men left were reduced to 300. Please note that the men that actually qualified for battle were less than 1% of the total number that came out for battle. This is a disaster!

From 32,000 men, who just by mere looks could have been qualified for battle now reduced to 300 men whose hearts actually followed the Lord wholly – this is incredible. This is a picture of the church today. I pray the Lord will not see you as a corpse, but as somebody that works and grows in the spirit.

You are the Devil's Enemy

Whether you believe it or not the devil does not see you as a friend. The Lord Jesus Himself said this in Mathew chapter 10 verses 16:

"Behold, I send you forth as sheep in the midst of wolves: be ye therefore wise as serpents, and harmless as doves."

The devil is aware of the declaration of war, so he is angry at the righteous every day. The moment you give your life to Christ the devil details his army of demons to stand on guard at your door. These demons watch your every move and wait for the convenient time to strike.

A man that has the life of God in him is the only one that can go to battle and return. They that wander out of the way of this understanding shall remain in the congregation of the dead, because they will continue to convince themselves that all is well with them until death finally encircles their necks with its fiery claws. It is important for you to know that the devil is a deceiver. He either flatters or flattens you. But

"..let him that thinketh he standeth take heed lest he fall". (I Cor. 10:12)

This fits the picture of a deceived man of God in Accra, Ghana. The Lord opened his eyes to see that a tree in front of his Church harbored strange birds. On impulse he ordered that the tree be cut down without any spiritual preparation. As soon as the tree landed on its side, the Pastor screamed. He placed his hand on his chest, with his eyes rolling wildly in their sockets and his mouth foaming with saliva, breathed his last breath, and passed on.

The enemy takes advantage of those who refuse to heed the counsel of God to use violence. Satan has been allowed to take over through neglect and carelessness. Where did the Pastor go wrong? He reduced a spiritual battle into level of the physical.

A family in our church in Lagos, Nigeria had a similar experience concerning the house they lived in. After much consultation with the revealer of secrets, the head of the family discovered that a tree in front of their house was a meeting point for witches who fly in as birds. He was inspired to place his hands on the tree and pronounce judgment upon it. As soon as he did, the tree dried up within three days:

"....Thus saith the Lord, In an acceptable time have I heard thee and in the day of salvation have I helped thee....." – (Isaiah 49 verse 8)

This connotes an answer to desperate prayers. They that cry receive help in time of trouble and they are preserved to do exploits as we further see in verse 8 of Isaiah 49:

"...and I will preserve thee and give thee for a covenant of the people, to establish the earth, to cause to inherit the desolate heritages;"

This same promise is beautifully articulated in the book of Isaiah chapter 58 verse 12 that they

"...that shall be of thee shall build the old waste places: thou shalt raise up the foundations of many generations and thou shalt be called, The repairer of the breach, The restorer of paths to dwell in."

This is the lot of the one who is willing to smash the gates of the enemy. And when they rise up to do so the following verse of scripture in Isaiah 49 verse 9 shall then be fulfilled:

"That thou mayest say to the prisoners Go forth; to them that are in darkness, Shew yourselves"

Here they have the privileges of setting the captives free from generations of imprisonment, and sadistic solitude. They lead those in darkness to light, help the helpless, and give hope to the hopeless. What a reward to a worthwhile labor when men go out to smash the gates of the enemy? The benefit of obedience is also encouraging. The one who sets free, and the people set free shall be at liberty to enjoy the benevolence of the Lord because:

"They shall feed in the ways, and their pastures shall be in all high places" (Is. 49:9).

Does this not confirm Psalm 23 verse 5? ***"Thou preparest a table before me in the presence of my enemies: thou anointest my head with oil my cup runneth over."***

Furthermore, The Isaiah 49 portion in verse 10 states that: ***"They shall not hunger nor thirst".*** This speaks of total deliverance from poverty and ***"...neither shall the heat nor sun smite them.."*** No more oppression.

Why? ***"..for he that hath mercy on them shall lead them, even by the springs of water shall he guide them."***

This is in line with Psalm 23 verse 2: ***"..he leadeth me beside the still waters"***

Inactivity Leads to Power Outage

Coming back to Psalm 82, what was God's reaction to those who refuse to fight? He simply disengaged them of power through the withdrawal of his grace. The privileges men used to enjoy just suddenly evaporated and He made a strong statement: ***"I have said, Ye are gods; and all of you are the children of the most high. But ye shall die like men.."*** (Ps 82:6-7).

This is a disaster and a terrible price to pay for inactivity. Men who had tasted power, who literally called down fire at will, who turned the world upside down are now to die like cockroaches. They are to die the death of the wicked. The power, which they used to enjoy and took for granted, has been withdrawn from them. They become the shadow of their former selves; extra-ordinary men that mere mortals now trample upon. The glory has departed and they are destined to die like ordinary men unsung. The covenant of grace has been taken away. Oh Lord! Let this not happen to any of your chosen that labors day, and night to see your kingdom come. Amen.

Rise up and fight

Having shared these facts with you it is time to wake up from lethargy, and put behind you those excuses, that have kept you under the oppression of the enemy for so long. When God arise all his enemies will scatter. Invite God to the battle and victory is yours. God is waiting for you to make the first move. He has promised to grant strength to the weak in time of war. Beyond this He has promised to equip you for continuous victory over your enemy.

"Behold, I will make thee a new sharp threshing instrument having teeth: thou shalt thresh the mountains, and beat them small, and shalt make the hills as chaff. (Is 41:15).

This promise is clear enough. Releasing yourself will ensure the fulfillment of this promise. Turn to Him and ask for

His help, he is willing to help you. Believe the Lord for he cannot lie, neither can he repent. Even more reassuring is what He expects you to do after the transformation. As we see in verse 16.

"Thou shalt fan them, and the wind shall carry them away, and the whirlwind shall scatter them: and thou shalt rejoice in the Lord and shalt glory in the Holy One of Israel."

No man will do the fighting for you. Note the words *"Thou shalt fan them.."* It is you that must do it. The solution is in your hands. Do not wait for the enemy to take the initiative. Make up your mind to be renewed in power and strength. God will surprise you. He will move in as you play your part and his: *"....wind shall carry them away, and the whirlwind shall scatter them...".*

Note that after the man's actions reduced the mountain to chaff and he began to fan them with 'warfare prayers', God released his wind to carry them away and his whirlwind completed the victory by scattering them. I assure you that like Humpty Dumpty they will never be put together again!

Do you want to be on the right side of power? Are you willing to enjoy victory through the grace given? That victory is yours if you say 'Yes I am willing to rise up to smash the gates of the enemy'. You will not only have that victory, but also rejoicing, because victory is automatically followed by the noise of rejoicing. Do you want to rejoice in the Holy One of Israel? Then rise up and fight!

FIERY DART PRAYERS

1.   O Lord I invoke the ministry of the hailstones to sweep away the refuge of lies from my village, town, city and nation in Jesus name.

2.   O Lord I invoke the ministry of the hailstones to sweep away the refuge of lies from my life, family or business in Jesus name.

3.   O Lord as I lay justice to the line, let the lines of my inheritance fall unto me in pleasant places and have a goodly heritage in Jesus name.

4.   Spirit of the living God I release the water of your word to overflow the hiding place of the enemy that they may be drowned like Pharaoh and his men of war.

5.   Father, I cancel today the covenant with death and agreement with hell, which the gates entered into on behalf of my community in Jesus name.

6.   Spirit of the living God, I cancel all evil covenants and agreements over my community and insist they will neither stand, nor come to pass in Jesus name.

7.   Father, I release the overflowing scourge of worded prayers and insist that the enemy shall not be hid from the scourge of my tongue in Jesus name.

8.   O Lord make the bed of the wicked shorter than that he can stretch himself on it, so that from today he loses his peace and rest in Jesus name.

9.   In the name of Jesus, I make the covering cloth of my enemy narrower than that he can wrap himself in it, so that from today he suffers from divine cold that will terminate him from the land of the living.

10.   In the name Jesus, I retrieve the keys to my destiny from whosoever is using them to manipulate my life for failure.

Chapter Nine
PREVAILING PRAYERS

"...Thy name shall be called no more Jacob, but Israel: for as a prince hast thou power with God, and with men and hast prevailed."
– *Gen 32:28*

Introduction

There is a need to rise up and fight the entities of darkness that have hindered us from entering into our possession in God and prevail. Jacob wrestled with God all night and he received a name change and destiny change. He equally received restoration in God, which accelerated divine blessing to begin to manifest all over him. The issue of restoration is very important and many should know that this is the platform upon which a man that is down must launch out. He must be willing to go all out for total possession of what he has lost to the kingdom of darkness – and this is one reason we are examining prevailing prayers.

Jacob's determination for breakthrough procured for him victory in prayer, name change, and divine blessings. Here was a homely man who circumstances and demand of the moment drew out the instinct of determination that caused him to prevail. Tommy Lasorda says "The difference between the impossible and the possible lies in a person's determination". Jacob made the impossible in his life happened because he was determined. Prayer power restored him to dominion in God. This cunning deceiver through prevailing prayer was visited by the very presence of God and:

"...as a prince hast thou power with God, and with men and hast prevailed."

The man Jacob did not only receive the mandate to exercise power in God, but also the ability to exercise power over men and has prevailed. Who did he prevail over after having power with God and with men? This man was given the liberty to prevail over the Kingdom of darkness. He was no more Jacob the cheat, because that yoke was broken that night.

Anyone who is unwilling to pray until something happens in his life will not prevail. This attitude must be ingrained in our thought processes. There should be no room for excuses, there is a need to rise up and go all out against the enemy to prevail. He is on the look out to take advantage, but if you place your hands on the plow without looking back you will prevail.

Resistance this counsel is an invitation to failure and disaster. Many have failed in life because they simply disobeyed the commandment of the Lord **"To watch and pray"**. Failure to heed this counsel will spell doom and if care is not taken the victim may not recover from the shock of recurrent defeats.

It is painful to see those who are expected to know, suffer cheaply in the hands of Satan, in spite of the price they paid in suffering with Christ. We saw an example, in the last few paragraphs of our discussion in the previous chapter. How God declared that the men who failed him would die as mere men. It is painful to note that this should be the portion of men who had paid the price of suffering with Christ, only to lose out in the last minute. They were to die cheaply without any remembrance of their once glorious past.

God's reaction to these men was predicated on His disappointment with them. God has invested so much in man and He expects returns in terms of fruits of service. The reason is that God depends on man to carry out His plan of evangelizing the world. He is looking for a man that will pray till his kingdom comes. This is the kind of person that can pray prevailing prayers.

Prevailing Prayer

Prevailing prayer is wrestling with God until you receive answer to prayer. It is manifest when a man tarries long and endures till God answers him. Daniel was such a man who wearied heaven with his persistent cries for twenty-one days and procured desperate answer, by overcoming the Prince of Persia through the power of his prayer. He held on fastidiously to the helm of God and refused to let go until God sent an Arch Angel to force change in the affairs of things.

We have heard several stories of numerous men who prevailed in prayer, but George Muller by my reckoning stood taller than them all. Here was a man who the account of his faith based praying drew the attention of heaven. He never for once turned back on a course of action in prayer. There was an account I read from a booklet prepared by Pastor Segun Osinaga about "Men Who Scared Hell By Prayers" Hear what was written about George Muller

".....**George Muller** was a great intercessor. He said, "I have been praying for sixty-three years and eight months for one man's conversion. He is not converted yet, but he will be! How can it be otherwise? There is the unchanging promise of Jehovah, on that I rest. "His prayers for that man were answered on Muller's burial day. No wonder he once exclaimed, 'Oh, how good, kind, gracious and condescending is the one with whom we have to do! I am only a poor, frail, sinful man, but He has heard my prayers ten thousands of times. "His prayer for that man was answered on Muller's burial day. No wonder he once exclaimed, "Oh, how good, kind, gracious and condescending is the one with whom we have to do! I am only a poor, frail, sinful man, but He has heard my prayers ten thousands of times."

What other example does one need to explain how to prevail in prayer? The man who must prevail in prayer must be willing to totally rely on God for strength. *"And they that do know thy name will put their trust in thee...."* (Ps. 9:10).

David knew this very well and hence attributed his success to God. He set aside his military skill or prowess and relied on direction from God. He waited patiently on Him, watching day and night for His help and God honored him by causing him to prevail over all his enemies.

Notice how he gave God the glory due to His name. He gave the victory to God without any strings attached: "... *thou hast subdued under me those that rose against me."*

Everyone who prevails in prayer will have testimonies to tell. That is why the Psalms of David are filled with the songs of rejoicing and testimonies. *"I will praise thee, O Lord, with my whole heart; I will shew forth all thy marvelous works (testimonies). I will be glad and rejoice in thee....."* (Ps. 9:1-2).

Why is this of particular interest? It is because of what God did in David's life as expressed by him in the later part of the chapter. Just like the gates of hell confronted the Lord Jesus Christ our Lord and Savior, they moved powerfully against David and almost killed him. We thank God that David was a man of prayer, praise and worship, who stood his ground to prevail in prayer. He lifted up his voice unto God, who is able to save His own from trouble and God in His infinite mercies intervened when David vehemently cried in (Ps. 9:13-14):

"Have mercy upon me, O Lord; consider my trouble which I suffer of them that hate me, thou that liftest me up from the gates of death: That I may shew forth all thy praise in the gates (public presence) *of the daughter of Zion: I will rejoice in thy salvation."*

The Secrets of Prevailing Prayers.

Prevailing prayer requires understanding certain secrets in God to enable one to prevail in prayer. It is not of him that wills but God that shows us mercy. The secrets unlock the door of prayer power, and make prevailing prayer a thing of joy to do. These form the bedrock of a person's prayer life, and determine whether he will prevail in prayer or not.

These secrets will open our heart and eyes to the mind of God on how to prevail in prayer. Please find them briefly enumerated below:

   i) **Relationship with God** – A sound relationship must exist between the man who must prevail in prayers and God. Such a relationship reveals the level of friendship that transpires between two longing souls.

   ii) **Pure Heart** – A pure heart is a fertile ground for God's words to grow and produce result in prevailing prayer. The praying person must as a necessity approach God with a pure heart and good conscience. (Ps 66:18)

iii) Holiness –Without holiness it is impossible to see Him, because he abhors the prayer of sinners and their sacrifices are abominations to Him. The praying person must therefore strive to be holy. (2 Cor. 7:1; Rom 6:19)

iv) Commitment to Prayer Request - The man that wavers or is unstable and cannot receive from God. God desires a man who must remain steadfast, single-minded, and committed to whatever prayer request put forward to God. He is one who can ask in faith with nothing wavering, such a man is the one that can prevail in prayer.

v) Close Walk with the Holy Spirit – To successfully achieve victory in prayer requires a good relationship with the Holy Spirit- specifically a close walk with Him.

vi) Know His Will in Prayers - A close walk will enable you to know God's will. You must cultivate this attitude in order to pray in His will and prevail in prayer.

vii) The Ability to Cry - **You** must be able to cry before him till he answers: ***"The righteous cry, and the Lord heareth, and delivereth them out of all their troubles."***

viii) Thanksgiving – You must be a person that offers willingly sacrifices of praise and thanksgiving. The key that opens the gate is thanksgiving and the one that opens His court is praise (Ps. 100:4)

ix) The Word of God

God cannot use a man in the place of prayer, except he sharpens himself through the study of the word of God: *" If the iron be blunt, and he do not whet the edge, then must he put to more strength..."* (Ecl. 10:10).

ix) Meditation

He must spend time in deep meditation and communion with the Lord in order to know which direction to channel his prayers because: *"The entrance of thy words giveth light; it giveth understanding...."* (Ps 119:130)

x) Fasting

It is important to seek the face of God and draw more strength from Him. The fast is for renewal of strength and direction.

Wait Till You See Result

God is looking for a man that will pray till his kingdom comes. This is very important and Job declared succinctly that: *"....all the days of my appointed time will I wait, till my change come."* (Job 14:14). Why did he decide for this option? It is simply because: *"If a man die, shall he live again?....."* (Job 14:14). Definitely no!

So it is important to wait in prevailing prayer and not die in suffering. Simeon prayed, waited on God *"...for the consolation of Israel..."* (Luke 2:25), and he prevailed. God had promised him and his unrelenting intercession helped to ensure that the Lord's Christ did come, and before his death too. When God's promise was fulfilled, he offered prayers of thanksgiving, blessed the child and prayed for God's release through death: "***Lord, now, lettest thou thy servant depart in peace, according to thy word***" (v29).

This was a real manifestation of grace. Man and God in a love relationship through fervent prayers. All he was telling God was **"Look, I have finished my assignment in prayers. I have done my part now you fulfill your promise by letting me die in peace**". He saw the salvation of Israel, because he obeyed and paved way for Him to come through ceaseless and selfless praying. Obedience and commitment to the prayer project gave Him a ticket to choose the time and kind of death.

Anna was another faithful intercessor, who prayed from her adolescence life till she was 84 years old. The Bible says she: "**.... departed not from the temple, but served God with fastings and prayers night and day**" (Luke 2:36).

It sounds incredible, but she must have done this probably for 60 years or more. She was also praying for the safe arrival of Jesus Christ. When she saw Him, she**: "*..gave thanks likewise unto the Lord, and spake of him to all them that looked for redemption in Jerusalem*" (v38).

How did she know that that little baby wrapped in cloths was the Messiah? It was by the revelation she received in the place of prayer. Joseph of Arimathae also faithfully waited in the place of prayer for the kingdom of God:

"Joseph of Arimathae, an honourable counsellor, which also waited for the kingdom of God, came, and went in boldly unto Pilate, and craved the body of Jesus" (Mark 15:43).

All the men mentioned above gave something in order to win Christ. They prayed and also sacrificed themselves and their substance. It is impossible to give God your substance if you have not given yourself to Him in prayer. Prayerless men are poor givers, because they cannot walk by faith, which is sustained by fellowship through prayer.

Praying men are givers, they give by unfeigned faith. We see this to be true about our brother Joseph the waiter. Through continuous waiting in the place of prayer he was convinced to provide a resting place for Jesus. Boldness came through much praying. They that wait upon the Lord shall renew their strength. While Joseph prayed, he received a divine revelation of the right place to bury the **rock** of our salvation, and the precious corner **stone** of our lives: *"...and laid him in a sepulchre which was hewn out of a rock, and rolled a stone unto the door of the sepulchre."* (v46).

When men pray they receive divine secrets that other men do not know. More importantly, God needs men that will pray till His promises are fulfilled here on earth. When the Son of man was to come, the services of Simeon and Anna were engaged to pray Him down. Joseph of Arimatthae, Mary Magdalene, Mary the mother of James, and Salome all prepared for his burial when He was to return to the right hand of the Father in glory, All these prayerfully waited and acted by the leading of the spirit to fulfill God's kingdom purposes.

FIERY DART PRAYERS

1.   Every veil covering my eyes be removed now!

2.   Spirit of the living God, Give me the ears of Samuel that I may hear divine ministrations from thy throne.

3.   All satanic blankets covering my eyes from advancing into my destiny be burnt with Holy Ghost fire.

4.   Spirit of the living God, Give me the eyes of Elisha that my eyes may behold your glory.

5.   Spirit of the living God, Give me the tongue of Elijah that my words will release fire from God's throne.

6.   I receive prayer power to prevail in prayer.

7.   I receive the wisdom of Joseph, that I may apply divine knowledge through godly wisdom.

8.   I receive the revelatory ability of Paul that I may be an effective intercessor that fights by revelation.

9.   I receive transfiguration experience as God gives me divine ability to dwell long on His holy mountain.

10.   I render impotent every spirit of complacency that has demobilized me from going forward.

Chapter Ten
HOW TO MAINTAIN YOUR VICTORY

"But the end of all things is at hand: be therefore sober, and watch unto prayer" - I Pet 4:7

Introduction

To achieve victory in life is always an uphill task. The maintenance of victory won is twice as difficult. Hence the need to maintain or sustain victory becomes paramount in the light of the above assertion. The grounds won in battle should not only be maintained, but be expanded by conquering more land. The ability to gain more grounds in life guarantees a person's upward move in life. However, this upward move can become a mirage if there is no backup plan to sustain it.

Many men have lost their cutting edge, not because they do not know how to move up. In actual fact, they have made many marks in getting to the top, but they have ended badly losing all they have gained in life because they do not know how to maintain their victory in Christ.

The Approach

The approach to adopt is summarized in the following verse of scriptures. A diligent intercessor should clinically follow the step-by-step guidance to maintaining victory. There is much wisdom in adhering to wise counsel. It is much more precious than gold:

"And the prophet came to the king of Israel, and said unto him, Go, strengthen thyself, and mark, and see what thou doest: for at the return of the year the king of Syria will come up against you." (I kings 20:22)

i) **Go.**

It is important to note that there is a coma behind the word 'Go'. This connotes an important instruction on its own, and not just a part of the sentence. The coma there reveals that the word 'Go' in itself is a command to take seriously. Having received your breakthrough you must go with the mind of being perpetually mobilized against the enemy and maintain your hold against him.

This is a mission that can only be made possible by maintaining close contact with the Holy Spirit. You must keep ascending spiritually with the determination that you will neither stop nor look back. The Lord Jesus sent forth his disciples and told them

"....Go ye into all the world, and preach the gospel to every creature" (Mk 16:15).

There must be a going forth to ensure and maintain your victory in Christ Jesus.

ii) Strengthen Thyself

This is a strategic counsel that if adhered to will guarantee continuous victory in the face of conflicts. The man that suffers defeat in battle, his strength is small. How does one strengthen himself?

You can do this through prayer, fasting, using the word of God, praise and worship and meditation. They that wait upon the Lord shall renew their strength. You may read details on fasting, prayer, praise, worship, and meditation in Chapters 4 and 5 of my first book *"Fighting Your Way To Victory – principles of victory over stubborn problems"*. However, please find them briefly enumerated below:

a) Prayer

What is Prayer? Prayer is communing with God, and committing into his hands ones desires and having an expectation of receiving his blessings. It is asking and receiving. It is a heartfelt communication between two spiritual lovers in a mutually beneficial covenant relationship. As a result, heavens know you and you know the power of heaven also, because, strength for victory comes through praying.

b) Fasting

Closely linked to prayer, and knowledge of the word is fasting. This is an indispensable weapon of war. God ordains it that a man should separate himself unto him: ***"Is this not the fast that I have chosen:.."*** (Is. 58:6).

God has chosen fasting to help us grow in the spirit and possess unusual abilities ordinary mortals do not have. Ideally a child of God should live a fasted life, where his first meal every day starts at 12.00 noon. One can eat only two meals a day, thereby giving one's breakfast to God as a holy sacrifice. This is beside the full fast he must have at least once a week.

c) The Word

The necessity of the word of God is mentioned in several parts of the bible. We see in II Timothy 2:15:

"Study to show yourself approved, a workman that is not ashamed"

How will you know if you do not spend time in the word of God. It is the truth that you know that can set you free. The word of God strengthens, enlightens, inspires cleanses, and delivers. The word of God is a lamp, fire, hammer, and sword that you can use in spiritual warfare.

d) Meditation

What is meditation? It is to ponder or think on God's word. When you ruminate on these words you establish the truth effectively in your spirit man. Meditation is the inward prayer of the heart. It is not blanking out your mind. Making your mind blank is treading on dangerous ground, as it will leave your mind open to other influence other than God's. This is satanic and is a usual practice with those practicing yoga, transcendental meditation and Chinese/Japanese martial arts just to mention a few. If you follow this path, you will open up a doorway to satanic oppression. Evil spirits will automatically take hold of your ignorance in passive meditation to take over your thoughts.

e) Praise, Worship and Thanksgiving

We have seen the importance of communing with God in the spirit and receiving answers to our prayers. Prayer as an activity however, is incomplete without thanksgiving, praise and worship. Thanksgiving is an expression of appreciation to God for what he has done, while praise is the exaltation of God for whom He is and what He had been doing in the lives of men. Worship or adoration is blessing God for His mightiness. Therefore there is a need to always:

"Enter into his gates with thanksgiving and into his courts with praise:.." (Ps 100:4).

iii) Mark

This is simply an advice to be either observant or vigilant especially in the area of one's dreams. The book of Psalm chapter 107 verse 43 counsels us to be observant:

"*Whoso is wise, and will observe these things, even they shall understand the lovingkindness of the Lord.*"

This verse points out that it is a wise man that will take time to observe these things. He is also the one that will understand the loving kindness of God after he had been delivered from the plot of Satan designed in the realm of the spirits, but revealed in dreams or by the move of the Holy Spirit in the conscious state of a man.

Dreams can be gateways to spiritual affliction. The powers of darkness raise satanic altars through dreams to afflict. This is sometimes revealed to the victim in dreams in order for him or her to stop the enemy from carrying out the affliction in real life. Everything you see in your dreams as you wake up, write the details down, and meticulously pray violently about each of the salient factors until you are sure of victory.

Only aggressive prayer can stop the enemy but many today have failed in this bid because they refused to heed this advice. There was the story of a woman, who acted like a fool. God revealed to her in a dream that her closest friend defecated on her head. She woke up telling herself, it could never happen, because her friend was a nice, well-cultured, or refined person. Secondly, she did not believe that she could be so foolish as to allow a thing like that to happen to her. She never bothered to pray about it.

Six months later, the devil struck, and her husband began to pick quarrels on almost everything she did. The man began to abuse her that she was giving off a bad odor. In less than a month thereafter, she was kicked out of the house and her closest friend through cunning intrigues moved in. She had been warned, but she did not understand the dream and was too complacent to find out. She wrongly perceived the dream and this became a costly mistake for her.

iv) See what thou doest

Be careful and do not take things lightly. Be watchful and alert unto prayers. The I Epistle of Peter 5:8 warns us: ***"Be sober, be vigilant; because your adversary the devil, as a roaring lion, walketh about, seeking whom he may devour."***

Note that in the story of the woman mentioned before, she was not sober and vigilant, and Satan took advantage of her weakness to devour her marriage. There are many in her category, who are too presumptuous, and therefore pay dearly for it. As a Christian you have to watch and pray, do not take things for granted, especially, when you observe some inexplicable obstacles in your life. The Lord will keep you, as you watch out diligently.

v) For at the Return of the Year the King of Syria Will Come Up Against You

This is a warning revealing the strategy of Satan, with regards to repeated assaults on its opponent in battle. It has been observed that, if he does not strike back immediately, he would wait till the third day, week, or month or when he notices a weak link in a person's life.

The Lord warns us that after a demon has been dislodged from a place, he will go and look for seven stronger demons to team up with him in order to re-occupy the place and the case of the person will be worse than the beginning. So be warned.

Prayer of Commitment/Decision.

Oh Lord, I (mention your name) commit myself today, to live a life of   prayers, where the things of the kingdom will reign supreme in my heart. Let the spirit of grace and supplication come upon me O Lord and make me a waiter that will achieve kingdom goals on your behalf. Then I shall remain dependable to commit prayer resources to divine economy as you use me. So help me God.

God Bless you. Now that you have finished praying take a further step by writing your decision on the first blank page of your Bible e.g. **I (mention your name) promise to pray for a minimum of two hours (or more if you choose) every day**. Sign the date and time that is the day, month, and year. I assure you, you will never be the same again from today. Amen.

FIERY DART PRAYERS

1. I receive grace to maintain my victory in Christ Jesus.

2. O Lord fill me with divine strength that I may continually overcome in battle.

3. I command all satanic blankets covering my eyes from seeing into the realm of the spirits be burnt with Holy Ghost fire.

4. Spirit of the living God, give me the eyes of Elisha that my eyes may see the plans of the enemy before they are executed.

5. Spirit of the living God, Give me the tongue of Elijah that my words will release fire from God's throne.

6. Spirit of the living God, Give me the prayer power of Daniel that I may prevail in the place of prayer.

7. Spirit of the living God, Give me the wisdom of Joseph, that I may apply divine knowledge through godly wisdom in sustaining my victory in Christ.

8. Spirit of the living God, Give me the revelatory ability of Paul that I may be an effective intercessor that fights by revelation.

9. O Lord! Let me have a transfiguration experience as you give me divine ability to dwell long on your holy mountain as I fast and pray.

10. O Lord I receive grace to minister praise, worship, and thanksgiving unto you in the name of Jesus.

Appendix

Notes

Chapter 2

1.	The Secret of Breakthrough Prayers Chapter 10 pg 171 by Rev. (Dr.) M. O. Aransiola.

2.	Elders At The Gate Chapter 5 pgs 31 & 32 by Rev. Mosy U. Madugba.

3.	Elders At The Gate Chapter 1 pgs 1 & 2 by Rev. Mosy U. Madugba.

4.	Elders At The Gate Chapter 1 pgs 2 & 3 by Rev. Mosy U. Madugba

Chapter 3

1.	The TELL Magazine (No. 17), April 23rd, 2001	with cover page title "FIRST LADIES ON THE LOOSE", The story quoted is entitled "A	Revealing Trend" and is on pg 66.

2.   The NEWS Magazine, July 31st, 2000 "QUOTES" column.

3.   The PUNCH Newspaper of April 6th, 2001 "News Behind The News" with the story entitled The 40 Wise Girls on PG 26.

4.   The PUNCH Newspaper of April 6th, 2001 "News Behind The News" with the story entitled The Phobia of a Governor's wife on PG 26.

5.   The PUNCH Newspaper of April 6th, 2001 "News Behind The News" with the story entitled The Phobia of a Governor's wife on PG 26.

References

i)   The gates of hell shall not Prevail Part I (Manual)

ii)   The gates of hell shall not Prevail Part I (Manual)

iii)   The Secret of Breakthrough Prayers by Rev (Dr.) M. O. Aransiola

iv)   Elders At The Gate by Rev Mosy U. Madugba

v)   The TELL Magazine (No. 17), April 23rd, 2001 captioned "FIRST LADIES ON THE LOOSE".

vi)   The NEWS Magazine, July 31st, 2000 "QUOTES" column.

vii)   The PUNCH Newspaper of April 6th, 2001 "News Behind The News" PG 26.

Other books by the Author

i)   Fighting your Way to Victory

ii)   Dealing with the Generation Wasters

iii) The Secrets of Prevailing in Prayer

iv)   The gates of hell shall not Prevail Part I (Manual)

v)   The gates of hell shall not Prevail Part II (Manual)

Contact

To Contact Taiwo Ayeni
For speaking engagements
Please write or call

email – taayeni@yahoo.com

Or

Rehoboth Bible Ministries Inc.
607 E. Abram, Suite One,
Arlington, Texas, 76010

Tel: 1- 972-742-7365
1- 972-602-1837
Fax:1-972-602-1837
Website:www.rehobothbministries

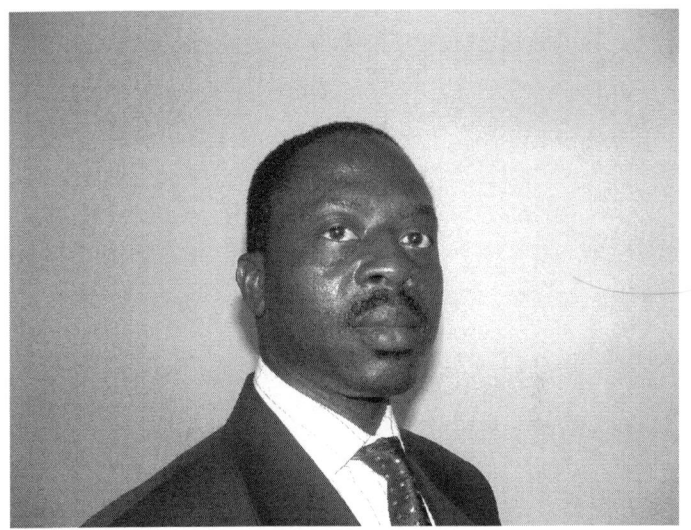

About the Author

Pastor Taiye Ayeni as he is fondly called, met with the Lord in his final year at the university of Lagos, Akoka, where he graduated with a Bachelors of Science combined honors degree in Mass Communication, Sociology, and Psychology.

Since knowing the Lord in 1983, he has been privileged to serve Him in various capacities. He is the Minister in Charge of Rehoboth Bible Ministries Inc, based in Arlington, Texas, USA and a Senior Lecturer at the Gethsemane Prayer Ministries International' Prayer School, with its headquarters in Ibadan, Nigeria.

He serves as the Minister in Charge of Prayer at Household Of Faith, of The Redeemed Christian Church of God (RCCG) Arlington, Texas, USA. He is presently in the

United States of America on mission for Christ, a graduate of the Advance Leadership and Pastoral School of Christ For The Nation's Institute (CFNI), Dallas. He is a graduate and member of the American Association of Christian Counselors (AACC); a mentoree of the prestigious LongRidge Writers Group in Connecticut and Chaplain intern at Methodist Dallas Medical Center, Dallas, Texas. He has widely traveled on speaking engagements within and outside the country in the course of ministry work.

He lives with his wife Dr (Mrs.) Abidemi Olubisi Ayeni and children, Rereloluwa (son) and Oreoluwa (daughter) in Grand Prairie, Texas.